ALL THIS SITTING IS KILLING YOU

All This Sitting Is Killing You

DR. PARLEY ANDERSON

Palmetto Publishing Group
Charleston, SC

All This Sitting Is Killing You

First Edition

Printed in the United States

ISBN-13 978-1-64111-590-2
ISBN-10: 1-64111-590-4

Sitting is more dangerous than smoking, kills more people than HIV, and is more treacherous than parachuting. We are sitting ourselves to death.

—James Levine, professor of medicine at the Mayo Clinic

Acknowledgements

I would like to acknowledge several individuals that have positively impacted my personal and professional development, and assisted in the organization and development of this book. First, and foremost, I would like to thank my parents Eldon and Karen Anderson. Thank you for taking a chance on me, for saving me, and for adopting me at the ripe old age of ten years. Without you two in my life, I truly do not know where I would be today. Your love, encouragement, and belief in me has enabled me to not only survive this life, but to grow, prosper, learn, thrive, and become the person and professional that I am today. I love you two with all my heart and soul. To Jim Mills: thank you for being my best friend. Not only are you a great friend, but you are an exceptional professional colleague as well. Also, I would like to send a big thank to Kayla Haugrud. Kayla was instrumental in assisting me with the research, development, and organizational layout of this book. I owe her an immense thank you in seeing my vision for this book become a reality. Next, I would like to personally thank Katelyn Elli Rose Welsh Photography and Jenny Kehoe. Katelyn is responsible for most of the photography in the book, and Jenny was the main fitness model used for many of the stretching and strengthening exercises displayed in this book. I love the professional photos and Jenny is truly an amazing fitness model. I would be remiss if I did not thank my amazing staff (especially Olivia Lane) as well as my professional colleague/business partner Michael Spevak. My staff (many of them pictured in this book) is made up of some of the most amazing and hard-working young people that I know. Thank you for everything you do for me. To Michael Spevak, thank you for being a great physical therapist, a great colleague, a great professional, a great mentor. But most of all thank you for being a great friend. Finally, I owe Erin Miller and Palmetto a big thank you for taking my manuscript and turning it into a true masterpiece (at least in my eyes). I am so happy with the final product that is this book.

Contents

Foreword

The impetus for writing this book first began several years ago while I was flying to Denmark for an international spine conference. I was browsing through an airline magazine and found an article titled "Sitting Is The New Smoking." The article discussed the negative effects on the body caused by sitting. About a year later, I attended an ancestral health conference in Berkeley, California. The main theme of the conference was how the development of modern civilization has resulted in a host of negative effects on the human body. One particular presentation was titled "Sitting Is Killing You." Once again, a host of negative effects that sitting has on the body were identified and discussed. Intrigued, I began doing my own research on sitting and how it affects our bodies and our minds. The results were truly disheartening. We as Americans sit for work, sit for play, and sit for most everything else. I call our current time the "Modern Age Of Sitting." Many medical and health practitioners have coined the term "sitting disease" in referencing the host of negative effects sitting has on the body. And the negative effects are not confined only to the body. A substantial amount of research also supports that sitting negatively impacts our mind as well. The good news is that many, if not all, of the negative effects of sitting on the body and the mind can be reduced, abolished, and prevented. "Motion is lotion, and rest is rust" is what I tell my patients. My main goal with this book is to give people easy and effective movement strategies to reduce, minimize, and eliminate the disease of sitting. A secondary goal is to provide a host of strategies and suggestions to not only survive but to truly *thrive* in this modern age of sitting.

Introduction

Video games, cell phones, cars, and televisions are just a few examples of technological advances contributing to the sitting epidemic plaguing the modern world. The average American spends 10–13 hours per day sitting, contributing to the unsettling statistic that 3.2 million deaths a year are related to physical inactivity.[7] A Harvard study found that 100 million Americans live with chronic pain related to sitting, with treatments and productivity loss costing around $635 billion. The Centers for Disease Control and Prevention found that in the United States, 7.6 million people list back pain as their reason for filing disability claims.[17] In addition, the CDC claims "worker illness and injury costs United States employers $225.8 billion annually." Apollo Hospitals found that sitting for six hours a day is equal to smoking more than a pack of cigarettes.

The sitting disease is the state of physical, mental, or emotional pain that results from being sedentary. Symptoms include neck and back pain, depression, obesity, and heart disease, and it may even lead to cancer. Fortunately, much can be done to reduce, eliminate, and reverse the plethora of health problems that the modern sitting epidemic has created in today's society.

This book is dedicated to providing readers with a better understanding of the effects of sitting on the body, and more importantly, providing specific strategies to combat, prevent, and reverse the myriad of problems associated with sitting. Additionally, readers will attain a better understanding of the many ways to improve their overall health and well-being.

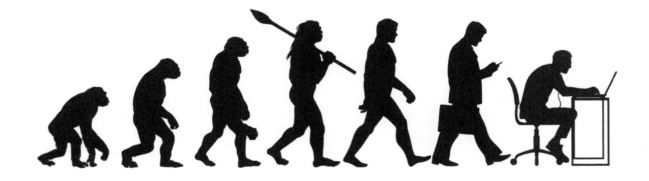

Medical Liability Release

Exercise and physical activity in and of itself presents with the possibility of suffering injury or pain. The information included in this book is not intended to substitute for professional medical advice. Rather it is intended to offer information in conjunction with your choice of health and/or medical provider. Please note that it is duty of the reader to take responsibility for his or her health, and for any and all advice they might receive from a medical or health specialist.

Scientific Support

In many places throughout this book, you will notice some sentences end with a small number after the period. These numbers reference scientific articles, journals, and publications that support the statements in the book. The details of each of these references can be found at the end of the book.

Chapter 1
The Sitting Problem

Work

On average, desk workers spend around ten hours a day sitting.[16] This accounts for 86% of American workers who utilize a chair in the office. As technology advances, so does the demand for desk work, increasing the number of individuals reporting chronic back pain and health issues related to a sedentary lifestyle. These health issues include diabetes, hypertension, depression, and muscle soreness.

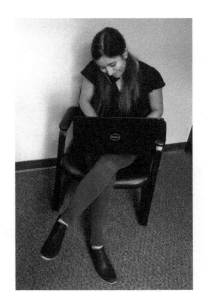

Unfortunately, in addition to the adverse health effects of prolonged sitting listed above, many individuals tend to sit with one leg crossed over the other, which causes more health issues and can lead to long-term damage. One article by the *Journal of Physical Therapy Science* explained that "sitting with the legs crossed may alter the weight-bearing or loads on soft tissues and muscles, resulting in unstable postures."[24] This sitting position can lead to improper alignment of the body, causing compensation to occur in order to maintain stability. An example of this is the way the pelvis rotates when forced into a cross-legged position, which can lead to problems in the lumbar spine region.

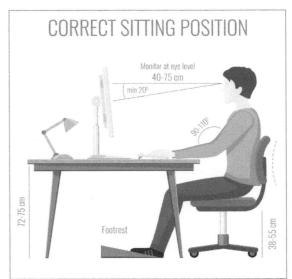

CORRECT SITTING POSITION

Monitor at eye level
40-75 cm

min 20°

90-110°

72-75 cm

Footrest

38-55 cm

The image to the right gives a good idea of the proper seated position while working at a desk. However, as the day goes on, it is likely that individuals in this position will begin to experience muscle fatigue in the areas responsible for keeping the body in proper sitting form, causing their posture to change and move into a more slouched postural position.

Cars

One study found that sitting in a car may be contributing to your heart problems. Men who spend over ten hours a week riding in a car had an 82% greater risk of suffering from heart disease than those who spent less time in the car.[16] The study found that "longer driving time was associated with higher odds of smoking, insufficient physical activity, short sleep, obesity, and worse physical and mental health."[25] In fact, the same study found that each hour spent in a car correlated with a 6% increase in obesity. When sitting in a car, try to mimic your posture to the young woman in the photo to the right. She is sitting up straight, keeping her arms in front, and looking straight ahead.

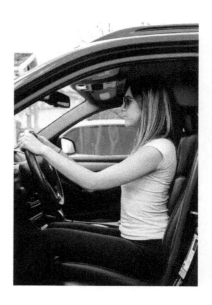

Video Games

In 2014, Nielsen explained that "players aged 13 and over spend more than six hours a week on any gaming platform."[18] In fact, 63% of households have at least one person who plays video

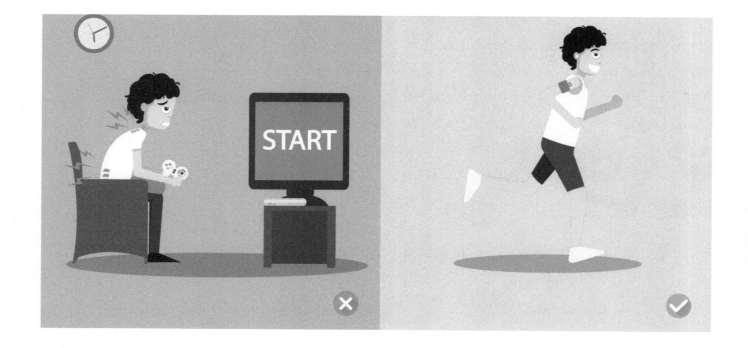

games regularly in the United States.[26] Surprisingly, only 27% of gamers are under 18 years of age, and 26% are 50 years or older, with 35 years being the average age of the gamer.[26]

It is no surprise, however, that those who play video games are typically seated. If added to the amount of time seated at school or work, riding in a car, and eating meals, those six hours may be taking away from time spent moving. Another factor to consider is the posture of the gamers. When your character, spaceship, or race car is winning the game, your posture may not seem nearly as pertinent until your back begins to ache and suddenly your reaction time to the game slows down.

Television

Whether sitting at home streaming your favorite show or at a theater to see the latest movie, much of the influence to sit comes from television. Statistically, adults watch on average more than five hours of television a day.[20] A study found that men who spend over ten hours a week watching television had a 64% greater chance of suffering from heart disease.[16] In fact, the *British Journal of Sports Medicine* found that "every hour of television watched may reduce our lifespan by an average of 21.8 minutes. Compare this health statistic to smoking a cigarette, which reduces our lifespan by an average of 11 minutes[17] Unfortunately, children are also highly affected by the sitting disease. A study done by *Preventative Medicine Reports* explained that children who watch television for more than three hours a day "have a 65% higher chance of being obese compared to children who watch less than one hour of TV per day."[19]

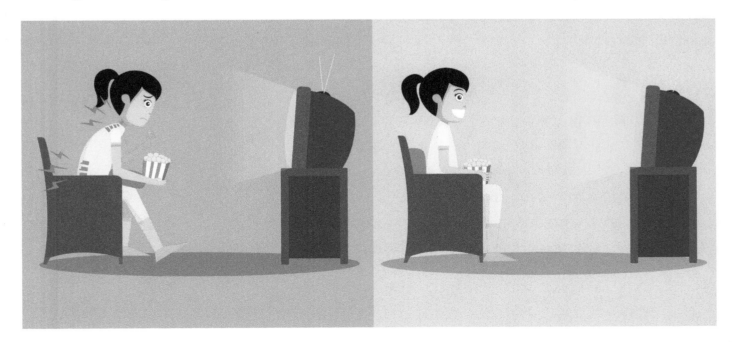

Chapter 2
The Effects of Sitting on Your Body

The body is very specific in how it likes to be positioned and how long it likes to be stationary. Any deviation from the body's normal demands can lead to negative symptoms and cause a great deal of stress both physically and mentally. Therefore, understanding the musculoskeletal system and its supporting parts is helpful in keeping the body in adequate condition. As the name implies, the musculoskeletal system encompasses the muscular system and the skeletal system of the human anatomy. This complicated system includes other structures of the body, such as ligaments, tendons, cartilage, joints, and tissues that all work together to maintain a healthy body. Unfortunately, this also means that when one part of the system has problems, other areas of the body are more likely at risk. This chapter will outline the impact sitting and sedentary behavior has on the musculoskeletal system.[1]

Bones

Bones are primarily made up of collagen and calcium. This combination accounts for the strength and flexibility of the bones to uphold the structure of the body. In order to maintain and build bone health, it is important to maintain a proper diet and incorporate strengthening practices into your daily routine. If

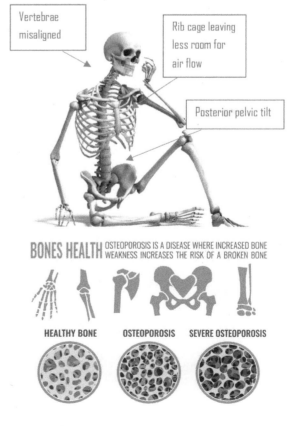

Vertebrae misaligned

Rib cage leaving less room for air flow

Posterior pelvic tilt

BONES HEALTH OSTEOPOROSIS IS A DISEASE WHERE INCREASED BONE WEAKNESS INCREASES THE RISK OF A BROKEN BONE

HEALTHY BONE   OSTEOPOROSIS   SEVERE OSTEOPOROSIS

ignored, the bones may become weak and unable to support the weight and movement of the body.

Prolonged sitting is associated with lower bone density, which can lead to osteoporosis due to an inhibition of bone growth factors. In fact, women can lose up to 1% of bone mass per year by sitting for more than six hours a day. In addition, misalignment of the skeleton can occur, leading to an abnormal curvature of the spine and an increased risk of chronic pain.

Muscles

Unused and weak muscles leave joints unstable and prone to injury and chronic pain. During sitting, glute, hip, back, and shoulder muscles weaken from lack of use. This muscle weakness affects posture and balance, thus making it harder to move freely. If weight-bearing muscles infrequently activate, adverse back curvature may become an issue. While there is a large number of specific muscles affected by sitting and inactivity, certain ones are affected more than others. These muscle regions include the hip flexors, abdominals, back extensors, legs, and shoulders. While sitting, muscle action is replaced by the support of the chair, leading to weakness. This weakness from sitting may also lead to loss of sarcomere length, and thus decrease the ability of the muscle to powerfully contract.

Structure of Skeletal Muscle

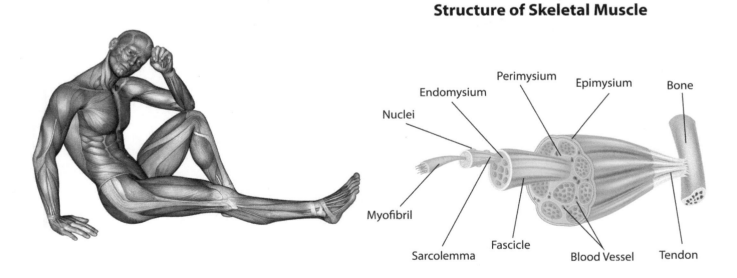

Tendons and Ligaments

According to the National Federation of Professional Trainers, "muscle strength is limited by the ability of the tendon to handle the force generated by the muscle."[27] Ligaments are then relied on to stabilize joints as the force is applied. Needless to say, tendons (which connect muscle to bone) and ligaments (which connect bone to bone) play important roles in the muscle contraction process. When a muscle contracts, it pulls on the tendon, which then pulls on the bone and movement occurs. Since these three structures work together to perform a task, such as lifting a weight, it makes sense that weakened muscles can lead to weakened tendons and ligaments. In addition, tendons and ligaments are not able to heal from injuries as fast as muscles due to their lack of blood supply.

When we sit for long periods of time, our muscles, tendons, and ligaments may become tight. Not only can this cause stiffness within the joints, it can also potentially lead to injury. With little elasticity within the muscles, tendons, and ligaments, a simple movement can cause a strain or tear. Unfortunately, a seated position compromises the muscles, tendons, and ligaments located all throughout the body, such as the neck, shoulders, spine, hips, and lower extremities.

Tissues

Similar to muscles, tendons and ligaments can either become excessively tight or excessively stretched as a result of prolonged sitting. Whether these tissues become too tight or too long (overstretched), it can lead to problems. As explained in the previous paragraph, muscles, tendons, and ligaments all work together to perform movement. Connective tissue is the key component in the formation of muscles, tendons, and ligaments. Connective tissue is composed of collagen and elastin fibers. Elastic fibers are responsible for the elasticity of the tissue, while collagenous fibers can be thought of as the strength component of connective tissue, containing mostly collagen.

Collagen accounts for three-quarters of the dry weight of skin and "is the most prevalent component of the extracellular matrix" of a cell.[77] This means that collagen is found in every individual's muscles, skin, blood, bones, cartilage, and ligaments. So obviously it's very important. According to Healthline, collagen is known to promote skin elasticity, hold together bones and muscles, protect organs, and provide structure to joints and tendons.[78]

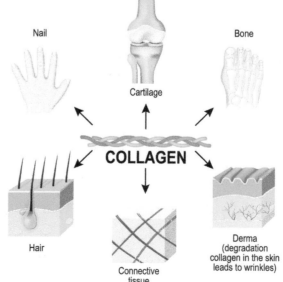

When the body is kept in a stationary position for long periods of time, such as sitting, certain muscles, tendons, and ligaments are being overstretched. Overstretching can make the tendons and ligaments more susceptible to injury, such as a tear. This sustained static stretching of tissues has actually proven to damage collagen by essentially weakening the fibers and causing atrophy. A review of muscle and tendon injury and overuse explains that "intermittent tendon loading generally promotes collagen turnover, healing, and remodeling processes" and should be done in replacement of static stretching.[103]

Cartilage

Cartilage is another important piece of the body that happens to be made up of connective tissue. It is found in many areas of the body, including joints in the shoulders, hips, knees, ankles, spine, fingers, and elbows. Cartilage is extremely important for proper joint movement and protection. An article published in the *Sports Health Journal* explains the role of articular cartilage, stating that its function is to provide a "smooth, lubricated surface for articulation and to facilitate the transmission of loads" with low friction.[38] In other words, cartilage must be able to protect bones from coming together by acting as a cushioned barrier. Unfortunately,

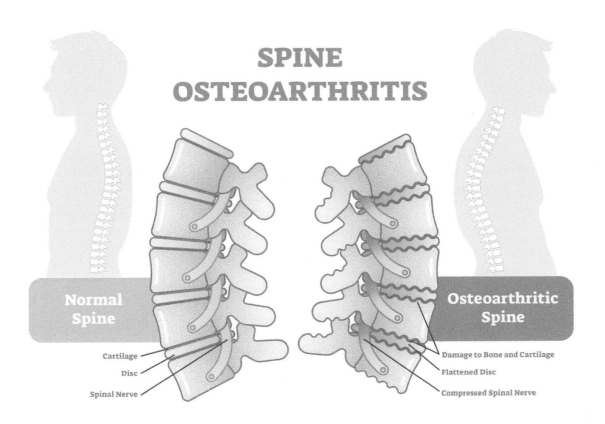

SPINE OSTEOARTHRITIS

Normal Spine

Osteoarthritic Spine

Cartilage
Disc
Spinal Nerve

Damage to Bone and Cartilage
Flattened Disc
Compressed Spinal Nerve

its ability to protect while allowing for smooth movement to occur is very difficult to replicate artificially, making surgical repairs difficult if damage has been done.

Joints

Joints are found where the ends of bones come together. They allow our body to move in three planes of motion known as the frontal, transverse, and sagittal planes. Joints can be immovable (synarthrosis), moveable (diarthrosis), or only slightly movable (amphiarthrosis).[56] In order to better understand how sitting affects our joints, it is important to start with the categories of joints. The main joints affected by sitting can be categorized into six groups: gliding, hinge, pivot, condyloid, saddle, and ball-and-socket joints. Gliding joints move against each other in a single plane, hinge joints move on one axis (such as flexion and extension), pivot joints allow for rotation, condyloid joints allow for circular motion, saddle joints allow for movements excluding rotation, and ball-and-socket joints can freely rotate on any axis.[56] Each of these joints can

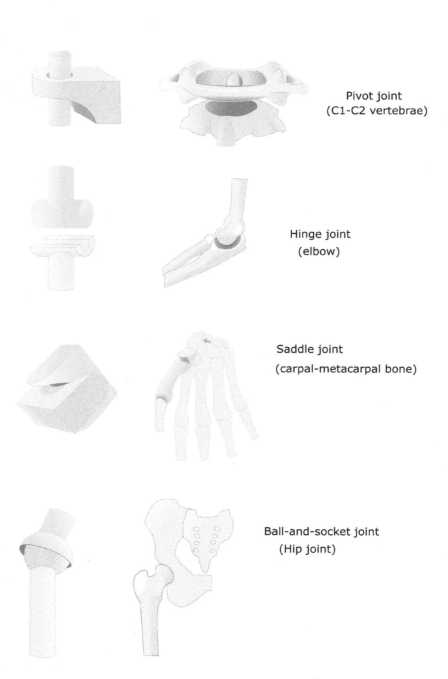

Pivot joint
(C1-C2 vertebrae)

Hinge joint
(elbow)

Saddle joint
(carpal-metacarpal bone)

Ball-and-socket joint
(Hip joint)

be referred to as synovial joints, which are characterized by a coating of articular cartilage on the ends of the bones. As previously discussed, articular cartilage lubricates the surfaces of bones and provides a smooth surface for movement to properly occur.

Postural Effects Of Sitting

Forward Head

Many working individuals rely on computers and laptops throughout the day. Depending on where the device is located in relation to their eyes, you may be leaning your head forward to see what is on the screen. This seemingly simple act of moving the head forward is only the first step toward developing bad posture. A forward head posture can be identified by extreme cervical spine protraction and flexion. This position is possible with the help of facet joints located between the vertebrae of the spine.

Rounded Shoulders

A forward head puts strain on not only the neck and upper back muscles but also on the shoulder joints and facet joints located throughout the spine. This postural stress naturally causes the shoulders to roll forward.

Increased Thoracic Kyphosis

The thoracic spine has a natural outward curve, known as the kyphotic curve. When in a seated position for a long period of time, this curve can become excessive, which is referred to as hyperkyphosis. In other words, this may give the image of being hunched forward.

Decreased Lumbar Lordosis (Flat Back)

Similar to the cervical spine, the lumbar spine has a natural inward curve called the lordotic curve. When seated for a long period of time, the angle of the inward curve can decrease (or even reverse), creating what can be seen as a flat back. The combination of hyperkyphosis and flat back are extremely detrimental to posture and overall health, which will be explained in the next few chapters of this book.

Tight Hip Flexors

Sitting activates the hip flexors of the muscular system. When muscles are forced to maintain the same length for an extended period of time without incorporating stretching or movement, they can become tight and uncomfortable. If the muscles become tight, they may become unstable and less mobile, leading to a higher risk of muscle strain. Muscle strain or tear often occurs when the muscles are not stretched enough for proper mobility and cannot sustain the lengthening of the muscle itself when forced to do so.

Inflammation

Living a sedentary lifestyle free of daily exercise and full of hours of sitting can even prove to affect inflammation of the body. Inflammation is an accessory to the immune system that alerts the body of harmful stimuli and addresses the problem through healing properties. The two types of inflammation are categorized as either acute or chronic. Acute inflammation is caused by "tissue damage due to trauma, microbial invasion, or noxious compounds" and "becomes severe in a short time." On the other hand, chronic inflammation is "slow, long-term inflammation lasting for prolonged periods of several months to years."[84] Common signs of inflammation include heat, pain, redness, and swelling. While inflammation is helpful in the process of identifying a harmful stimulus, a problem emerges when the inflammation persists. If the invader has not been completely eliminated or the "helper" T cells continue the invasion to fight the issue, inflammation will be present.[85] Chronic inflammation has been known to cause diseases such as diabetes, obesity, arthritis, and cardiovascular disease.

While prolonged inflammation can be detrimental, there are preventative measures that can be taken to ensure a well-working immune system. Some studies have found that an increase in physical activity has the ability to lower inflammation in the body. The energy expenditure experienced through exercise

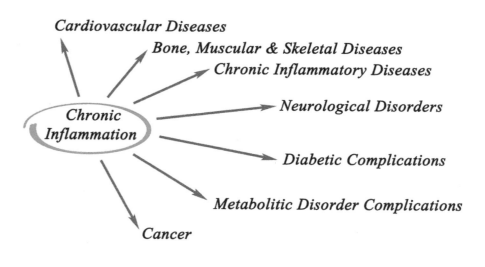

"lowers multiple pro-inflammatory molecules and cytokines independently of weight loss."[84] One study evaluated 4,289 people over a ten-year period and found that those who followed standard physical activity recommendations for cardiovascular health (2.5 hours per week of moderate to vigorous physical activity) maintained lower levels of inflammatory markers than those who did not follow proper exercise guidelines.[86]

Diet is another factor that may affect an individual's risk of developing chronic inflammation. Based on an article from the peer-reviewed medical journal *Psychosomatic Medicine*, diet, stress, and inflammation are all interrelated. Certain key factors, such as autonomic nervous system activity, oxidative stress, activation of a DNA transcription protein, and metabolic responses to food caused by diet and stress have the ability to significantly increase inflammation in the body. According to the article, diets that are "high in refined starches, sugar, saturated and trans-fats, and low in omega-3 fatty acids, natural antioxidants, and fiber from fruits, vegetables and whole grains" are known to promote inflammation.[101]

Foods that Decrease Inflammation   **Foods that Increase Inflammation**

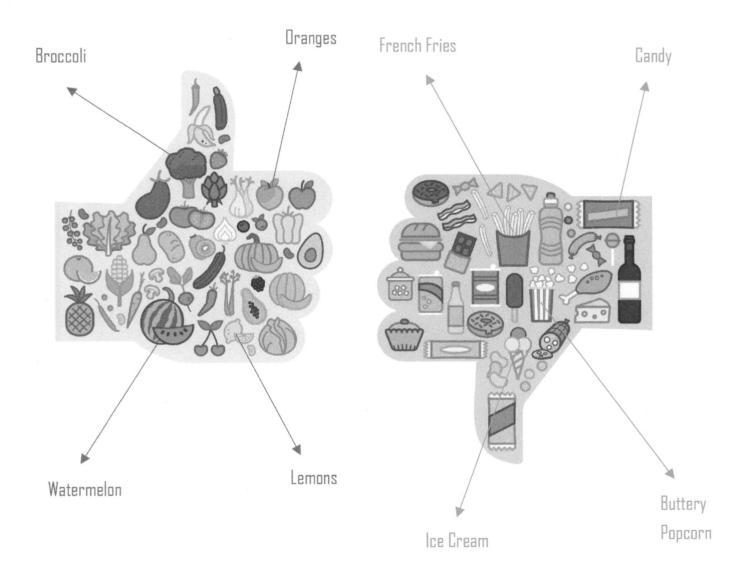

Broccoli   Oranges   French Fries   Candy

Watermelon   Lemons   Ice Cream   Buttery Popcorn

Chapter 3
Sitting and Longevity

Sitting has been shown to drastically impact areas of health such as cognitive function, blood circulation, heart health, mental health, metabolism, and aging. This chapter provides an overview on how these areas of health are affected by long-term sedentary behavior.

Cognitive Function

Movement of the body is done with the help of motor neurons, which allow the brain to tell the muscles what and how to move. Studies have shown that there is a connection between living a sedentary lifestyle and declined intellectual function. When muscles are told to activate, blood carries oxygen throughout the body to assist in the movement, as shown in the image below. However, when muscles stay still, brain function slows. A study done by Michigan State University proved that students who spent an excessive amount of time sitting had a difficult time retaining information when compared with their active counterparts.[10] A separate study found that breaking up sitting time with light-intensity activity may improve brain health by "maintaining glycemic control."[3] Glycemic control involves sustaining blood glucose levels within normal range of the individual, which can prevent diseases such as diabetes and hypo- or hyperglycemia from occurring.

Brain-derived neurotrophic factor (BDNF) is essential for survival of cognitive function, playing a role in survival, growth, learning, and memory.[11] When

MOTOR NEURON

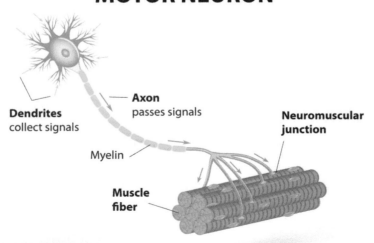

Dendrites
collect signals

Axon
passes signals

Myelin

Muscle
fiber

Neuromuscular
junction

an individual remains sedentary for much of their time, this factor is compromised, leading to decreased concentration and increased forgetfulness. In a study published through the *Journal of Sports Science and Medicine*, a 13% decrease in BDNF serum was found in sedentary individuals.[12] The same study found increased levels of BDNF as a result of physical activity.

To sum up conclusions presented through the research, cognitive function can be negatively affected when an individual spends prolonged periods of time sitting.

Blood Circulation

When sitting for long periods of time, blood circulation slows and can cause blood to pool in the legs and feet, "which can lead to varicose veins, swollen ankles, or even dangerous blood clots like deep vein thrombosis (DVT)."[16] Simply put, varicose veins happen when blood pressure increases in the superficial veins of the lower extremities. This happens when the valves in the veins become weakened or damaged from expanding due to the increased pressure from sitting. Instead of pushing nutrient-rich blood up and to the heart, blood pools in the legs.[46]

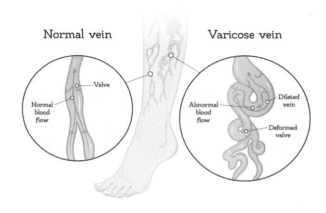

If blood clots form in the deeper veins of the legs, such as when DVT occurs, there is a high risk of the clot traveling to the brain and possibly causing a cerebrovascular accident (also known as a stroke). If an artery gets blocked by a blood clot, two major problems may occur. One is that a pulmonary embolism can occur in which the clot travels to the lungs.[46] The second is a myocardial infarction (also known as a heart attack) in which the clot travels to the heart.

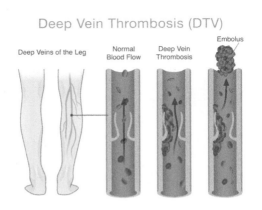

Heart Health

Prolonged sitting increases the risk for cardiovascular disease and doubles the risk if seated for over eight hours a day. In fact, 30% of ischemic heart disease cases are associated with a sedentary lifestyle. When a sedentary person burns less fat and blood circulation is poor, "there is an increased chance of fatty acids blocking the arteries in the heart." This blockage then influences the individual's risk of high cholesterol and blood pressure levels which can lead to cardiovascular disease. In fact, after just two hours of sitting, good cholesterol drops 20%.

Mental Health

Sitting for six or more hours a day increases the risk for anxiety and depression. According to a study conducted by BioMed Central, individuals who sit for long periods of time each day show decreased physical activity, sleep problems, poor psychological well-being, decreased academic behavior, and lower self-esteem and prosocial behavior.[15] The study also explains that "engaging in screen-based entertainment, such as video-gaming, has been shown to increase the arousal of the central nervous system, which could potentially lead to increased levels of anxiety."

Serotonin, dopamine, and norepinephrine are chemical neurotransmitters in the brain that act as messengers. Typically, when these chemicals are released, the mood of the individual is altered, giving off feelings such as relaxation, motivation, and determination. Many scientific journals have been published on the positive effects of exercise on the release of serotonin, dopamine, and norepinephrine; explaining that exercising stimulates the release of these neurotransmitters while being inactive shows little to no release. An individual suffering from depression may have an inadequate release of the euphoric chemicals and thus may not feel motivated to exercise.

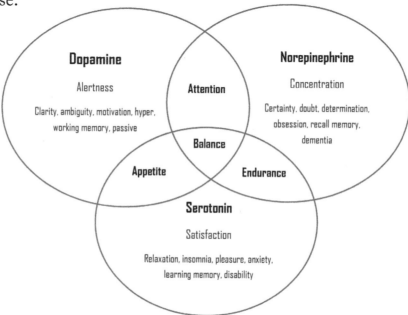

Metabolism

Metabolism is the sum of all chemical processes that occur within the body to sustain life. A person's metabolism is responsible for maintaining proper function of the organs, repairing cells, and digesting food. In order to maintain these processes, the body requires energy, specifically a basal metabolic rate (BMR).[47] BMR is the number of calories required to keep your body functioning at rest. Sitting reduces the production of enzymes that metabolize food and break down fat by 90%. In fact, spending 30 minutes in any fixed position starts to inhibit metabolism, and four hours of inactivity causes the near shutdown of an enzyme that controls fat and cholesterol breakdown. A sedentary individual typically has more fat cells, which require less energy to breakdown, whereas active individuals tend to have more muscle cells which require more energy to breakdown. With more energy needed, the active individuals will have a faster metabolism (higher BMR) than those who live a sedentary lifestyle.[47]

According to the Cleveland Clinic, metabolic syndrome is "a collection of heart disease risk factors that increase your chance of developing heart disease, stroke, and diabetes." This is a growing concern among a technology-driven society such as the United States, with one in five Americans showing signs of the syndrome. In fact, metabolic syndrome affects more than 40% of people in their 60's and 70's.[58] As we've already discussed, sitting is a risk factor for heart disease due to its negative influence on blood pressure and its correlation with sedentary or inactive behavior.

This diagram shows the risk factors that can lead to metabolic syndrome. According to the National Heart, Lung, and Blood Institute, at least three out of the five risk factors listed are required for an individual to be diagnosed with metabolic syndrome. [59]

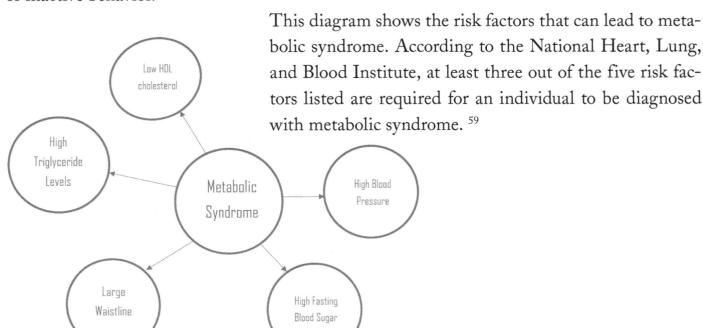

Telomeres

Telomeres act as a protective cap on the end of DNA-carrying chromosomes and prevent the loss of DNA during cellular divisions. A good analogy for a telomere is to think of your shoelaces and the "caps" at the end of the shoelaces that hold the strands together. Telemeres act as that protective "cap." at the ends of chromosomes. As cells divide throughout a person's lifespan, the protective cap shortens. The American Public Health Association, with the help of Xue et al., found that "because telomeres shorten with cell division or damage, telomere length can act as a quantifiable proxy of biological aging and damage accumulated across a lifespan."[20] In other words, telomeres (based on their length) offer a reasonable measure of an individual's physiologic age.

As it turns out, the length of these chromosomes can be altered based on certain factors, including living a sedentary lifestyle. The study by Xue et al. also found that "each one-hour increase in television watching was associated with a 72-base-pair decrease in mean telomere length," which "translated to a difference of approximately 1.2 to 1.8 years in biological age"[20] This same study also found similar associations in telomere length when comparing smokers with nonsmokers. Another factor of unhealthy shortening of telomeres includes oxidative stress and lack of physical activity. An article written by the *Open Access Impact Journal* explains that "Excessive Reactive Oxygen Species (ROS) production can cause oxidative stress in cells,

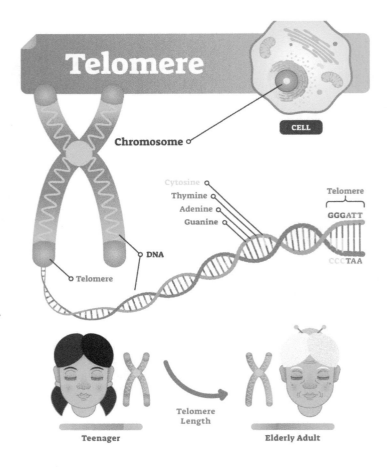

tissues, or organs, leading to DNA damage and senescence or apoptosis."[23] The article goes on to explain that regular exercise has been shown to lower oxidative stress and would, therefore, be beneficial in the protection of telomeres. Results from a study outlined in the same article found moderate physical activity to be associated with longer telomere length.

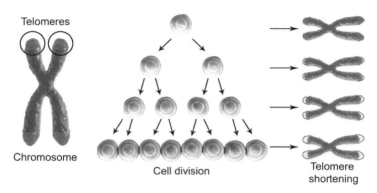

You may be wondering, "Can we lengthen telomeres?" Some research exists to support the case that lengthening telomeres is possible through the help of telomerase, the enzyme that replaces the lost telomere length by adding nucleotides to the ends of chromosomes in order to increase the stability of the DNA-carrying structures.[22] The theory is that if we can increase the amount of telomerase in our system, we have the ability to lengthen our telomeres and, therefore, be less likely to suffer from health issues. Currently, there are dietary supplements that supposedly promote the creation of telomerase.

Although the theory seems tangible, it may not be wise to supplement pro-telomerase activity. Dr. Harriet Hall confronts the telomerase-promoting supplement Product B and explains that the supplement may be more dangerous than helpful. For example, telomerase is active in cancer cells, which are known to divide rapidly and uncontrollably. In fact, as Dr. Hall puts it, "We don't want cancer cells to live forever…drugs that reduce telomerase activity are being investigated as cancer treatments."[21]

There is currently a lack of research on promoting and inhibiting telomerase activity. However, much research has proved that a healthy lifestyle, including diet and exercise, slows down the telomere shortening process. Another article written by the *Journal on Aging* explained that "obesity, insulin resistance, and cardiovascular disease process have all been linked to shorter telomeres."[21]

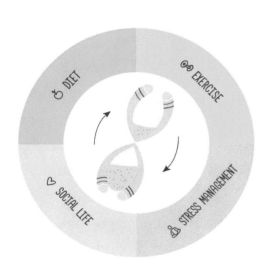

LIFESTYLE CHANGES
MAY LENGTHEN TELOMERES

Chapter 4
Sitting and Your Cervical Spine

For many individuals, computers, cell phones, and tablets are relied on in order to get work done and communicate. Unfortunately, much of the time spent utilizing these technologies is done in a seated position. And if the screen of the device is not up high enough, we may have to lower our heads in order to see properly, which can damage and/or strain the cervical vertebrae. The more we tilt our heads forward, decreasing the angle of the vertebral joints, the more force we exert on our cervical spine. If this force is applied over an extensive period of time, the cervical spine may encounter problems. Many chronic neck issues and injuries arise from prolonged sitting. For example, one study found that 81% of individuals who live sedentary lifestyles reported neck or shoulder pain symptoms.[28] Fortunately, much of the chronic neck pain associated with poor posture can be understood and prevented. This chapter includes an overview of the components of the cervical spine and issues related to improper positioning of the cervical spine region.

Cervical Anatomy

Between each vertebra in the spine are shock-absorbing, flexible, intervertebral discs that prevent the vertebrae from rubbing together while simultaneously allowing for movement to occur. These discs contain a nucleus pulposus wrapped within an annulus fibrosis. Since 66% - 86% of the nucleus pulposus is made of water, it is responsible for the majority of the spine's flexibility.[8] The discs have the ability to "counteract forces that act to

Anatomy and physiology of the vertebrae

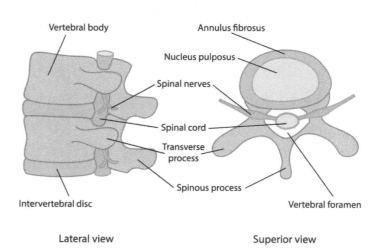

Vertebral body
Annulus fibrosus
Nucleus pulposus
Spinal nerves
Spinal cord
Transverse process
Spinous process
Intervertebral disc
Vertebral foramen

Lateral view
Superior view

18

lengthen or compress the spine" and "separate the vertebrae to allow spinal nerves to exit intervertebral foramina."[8] Since nerves can often be the source of pain or discomfort throughout the body, it is important that these discs operate in a way that allows space for the nerves to exit. Since discs connect vertebrae together, they are considered joints of the spine.

Unhealthy Cervical Positions

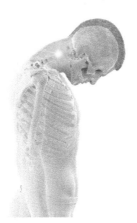

When the head is constantly placed in a forward leaning position where the individual is looking down (such as reading a book while sitting in a chair), the added weight can cause the vertebrae to push the discs posteriorly (toward the back), creating a high risk for bulging disc, herniated disc, and degenerative disc disease to occur.

These same risk factors may present in instances in which the head is leaning forward but looking ahead (such as while watching television sitting

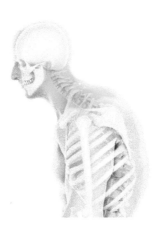

forward). In this case, the discs are forced anteriorly (toward the front) as pressure is increased on the back of the discs. Another example of this occurring is sitting too close to the big screen at the movie theater and having to look up.

Neck Pain and Balance

Whether neck pain occurs from poor posture or an injury, balance is at risk of being compromised. A study done by J. B. Chester in 1991 found that severe neck pain can be associated with decreased balancing ability. The American Posture Institute further explained that "neck trauma and vestibular impairment contributes to abnormal biofeedback, the function of maintaining body balance." The torque, which is a twisting force that causes rotation, might be changed to maintain posture which "is associated with reduced balance controlling ability."[61] In addition, neck pain or inflammation can reduce sense in the joints and can cause proprioception inadequacies, leading to improper balance. The term "cervicogenic dizziness" refers to dizziness/vertigo symptoms that result from trauma/pathology of the cervical spine.

Pinched Nerve

With the combination of forward head posture and forward shoulder posture comes a high risk of nerve compression. Nerves run throughout the body and are in constant communication with the brain. This means that they always have the ability to send signals of sensations to and from the brain. When the body is morphed into a position that is anatomically incorrect, nerves can be at risk for compression. Nerve compression or pinching occurs when certain structures, such as an intervertebral disc presses on a nerve. In this case, sensations of numbness, tingling, and even pain may occur.

The median nerve is especially at risk for compression during forward head posture paired with forward shoulder posture. The median nerve originates from the brachial plexus and runs down the arm. It is often associated with carpal tunnel syndrome but can be compressed at any point from the axilla (shoulder region) to the wrist. When the shoulders move forward, nerves are given less space to slide. If compression of the nerve is too great, the nerve can demyelinate, cutting off communication to and from the brain and even causing muscle inactivation. Once the nerve is damaged, repair can be difficult or even impossible.

Cervical Radiculopathy

Sometimes, nerve roots that emerge from the cervical region become compressed, leading to what is called "cervical radiculopathy." This condition can send sensations of pain, numbness, and tingling from the neck to the arms, upper back, chest, and shoulders. Compression of the nerve roots can happen when disc problems become evident, such as disc herniation, bulging, and degeneration. A common cause of disc problems is poor posture. This is due to the pressure of the vertebrae pushing the disc toward the spinal cord and thus compressing the proximal nerve root.

One way to combat the effects of cervical radiculopathy is to practice proper posture, paying close attention to maintaining cervical lordosis. One study was done through the *Journal of Physical Therapy Science*, in which a 31 year old male with cervical radiculopathy was treated with "cervical extension exercises, cervical extension traction, and spinal manipulative therapy."[96] After 40 treatment sessions over 17 weeks, the individual reported "alleviation of upper arm weakness and neck pain" and experienced significant reduction in forward head posture accompanied with restoration of cervical lordosis. One year later, reports showed the individual had maintained proper posture that had been established through the treatment sessions.

A Cervical Epidemic: Text Neck

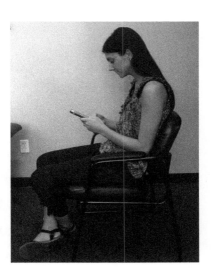

While the ability to communicate through written cell phone messages (texts) arguably been proven to enhance productivity, it has also introduced a concept referred to as "text neck." Text neck, coined by Dr. Dean L. Fishman, is "a term used to describe the neck pain and damage sustained from looking down at your cell phone, tablet, or other wireless devices too frequently and for too long."[30] So how often do we actually keep our heads in this detrimental position? An article written by Kenneth Burke through a website called Text Request outlines alarming statistics about the cell phones that have taken over the world.[29] These statistics include the following:

- The number of monthly texts sent increased more than 7,700% over the last decade (Statistic Brain).

- Over 560 billion texts are sent every month worldwide (Statistic Brain).

- More than 4.2 billion people text worldwide (MBA Online).

- 81% of Americans text (Paw Research Center).

- America is responsible for approximately 45% of the world's text volume (CTIA and Statistic Brain).

- Americans text twice as much as they call, on average (Nielsen).

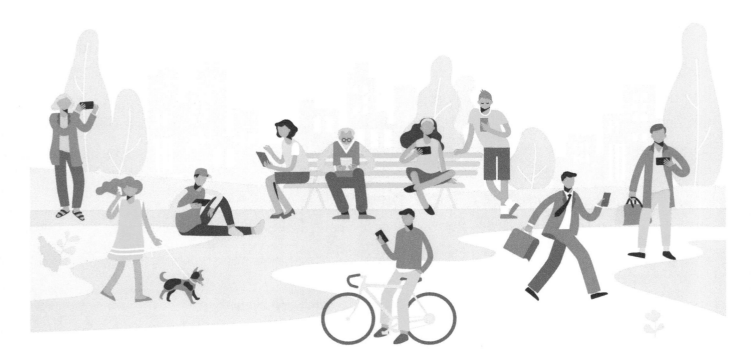

Another article outlines a systemic review on text neck and explains that 79% of the population between the ages of 18-45 years old have their cell phones with them at all times, with only two hours of their walking day spent without the phone in their hand.[42] As the population within the 79% statistic grows older, and the age of children given phones decreases, the text neck epidemic is on track to becoming a significantly more problematic issue troubling medical professionals today, and into the future.

Forward Head Tilt

While texting, the cervical and thoracic regions of the spine are forced to maintain a forward flexed position, adding weight to the spine and creating possible risk factors for future neck

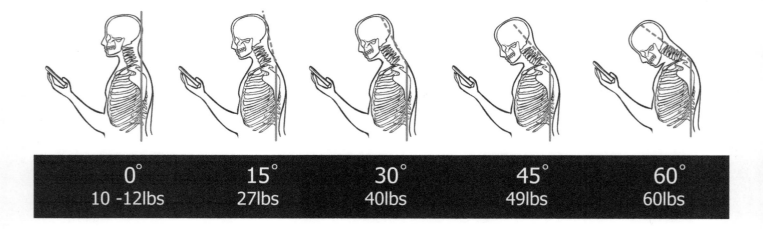

Smartphones are ruining our postures and stiffening our necks

0° 10 -12lbs	15° 27lbs	30° 40lbs	45° 49lbs	60° 60lbs

injuries. An article written by the *Imperial Journal of Interdisciplinary Research* explains that "when the head tilts forward at 15 degrees, the forces on the neck surge to 27 pounds, at 30 degrees 40 pounds, at 45 degrees 49 pounds, and at 60 degrees 60 pounds."[31] The article goes on to address the concerns of children keeping their head in a forward flexed position "since their heads are larger in relation to their body size than adults." Some symptoms of text neck include sharp pain, soreness, stiffness, muscle spasms, radiating pain, weakness, numbness, and headaches. If these symptoms persist, they can lead to injuries. Examples of the negative effects related to text neck are explained in the next few pages.

Flattening of the Spinal Curve

The cervical spine has a lordotic (inward) curve, similar to the lumbar spine. When kept in a forward flexed position for prolonged periods of time, such as when looking down at a cell phone, the creation of a flat neck may occur. This is known as cervical kyphosis. Cervical kyphosis is dangerous because, as mentioned earlier, there is increased pressure placed on the discs located between the vertebrae, which may cause the discs to bulge or become dehydrated.

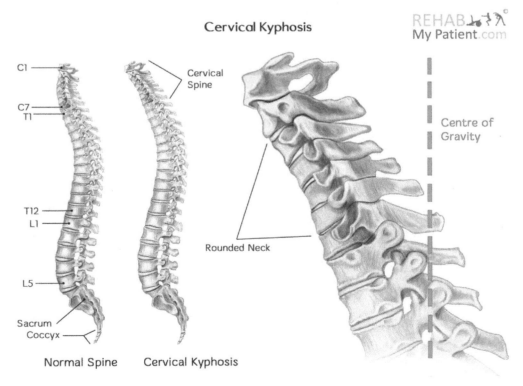

Picture from rehabmypatient.com

Spinal Degeneration/Arthritis

When the head is held in a forward flexed position for a period of time, the ligaments in the back of the neck stretch to allow for movement. Over time, the ligaments lose their elasticity after being overstretched, causing the vertebrae they support to lose stability and put more pressure on the discs. With increased pressure on the facet joints, the discs begin to lose height, causing there to be less of a shock-absorbing cushion for the vertebrae to sit on and more of a risk for collapse or inflammation of the discs. When the discs become too dehydrated, the bony vertebrae may begin to rub together, leading to symptoms of arthritis and degeneration.[34]

Disc Degeneration/Bulge/Herniation

If the discs become compressed, as mentioned above, the inner part of the disc, called the nucleus pulposus, may protrude out into the spinal canal, compressing the nerves that exit between the vertebrae. The disc can bulge out and cause problems but does not become a herniated disc until the inner nucleus pulposus completely breaks through the annulus fibrosis (hard outer covering of the disc) and pushes into the spinal canal. When this happens, symptoms of pain, numbness, tingling, or weakness may appear.[35]

DISC DEGENERATION

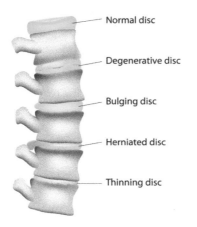

Normal disc

Degenerative disc

Bulging disc

Herniated disc

Thinning disc

Nerve Damage

When the spine experiences degeneration, disc herniation, or disc compression, the nerves may start to be affected. Many of the injuries associated with text neck can lead to compression of the nerves that run through the spinal column, which can create undesirable effects.

Muscle Damage

When the head is in typical texting position, meaning forward flexed, certain muscles are strained, tightened, and overstretched. This can lead to damages of those muscles that are now overactivating or underactivating. When a strain occurs, the muscle or tendon tears, typically causing pain, spasms, and tightness in the area. In addition to muscle strains, headaches can also be a result of excessive texting.

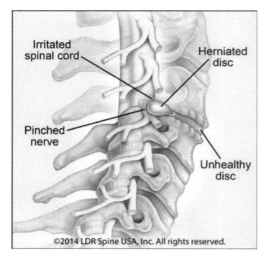

Irritated spinal cord

Herniated disc

Pinched nerve

Unhealthy disc

A tension headache is a concern among those with text neck symptoms. This happens when the muscles behind the neck tighten to a point of irritation and discomfort, causing pain in the form of a headache.[42] The American Posture Institute explains that tension headaches are the most frequently occurring headache disorders seen in adults. They explain that "population-based studies indicate one-year prevalence rates of 38.3% for episodic tension headaches."[61] A study done by Fernandes-de-las-Peña's in 2005 proved that there is a correlation between higher forward head posture and the frequency of tension headaches.[61]

Upper Crossed Syndrome is another condition that can occur from bad posture, characterized as deformities of the muscles in the neck, shoulders, and chest. An article through Healthline explains that the trapezius and levator scapulae are most often affected when they become strained and overactive, while the pectoralis major and minor (located at the front of the chest) become tight and shortened.[43] While these muscles are overactive, other muscles in the area are weak and underused. When the overactive and underactive muscles overlap, the upper crossed syndrome occurs.

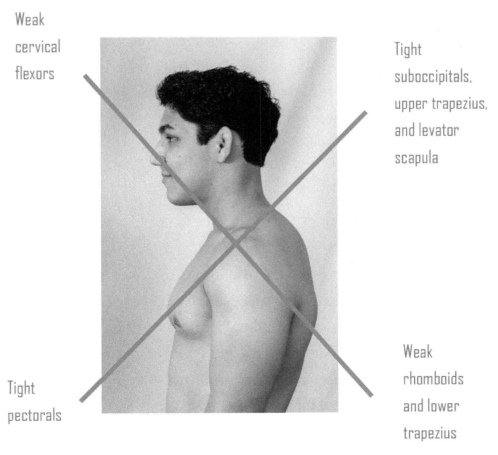

Weak cervical flexors

Tight suboccipitals, upper trapezius, and levator scapula

Tight pectorals

Weak rhomboids and lower trapezius

Dowager's Hump

Forward head posture has been proven to round the shoulders forward due to the stress loaded on the muscles and ligaments, creating an excessive kyphotic curve in the upper back. The book *Deskbound*, written by Dr. Kelly Starrett, explains that "in an attempt to even out the forward weight distribution of your head, your body will create a fat deposit under the skin of your upper back." In doing so, the body is straining to extend the head back to its healthy position by pulling on the overstretched connective tissue on the upper back. The fat deposits can lead to the creation of a rounded protrusion, known as a dowager's hump.

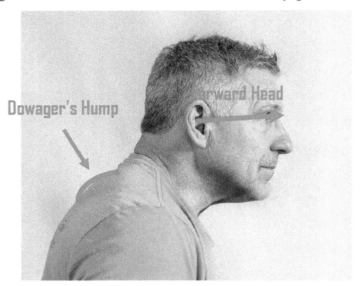

This fatty formation, if excessively large, can lead to painful and detrimental health problems. As mentioned above, the hump can worsen as the spinal ligaments continue to stretch, putting pressure on the spinal column. Sometimes, osteoporosis can be a cause of dowager's hump due to a weakening of the bones and a loss of bone density, causing the spine to easily bend.[60] When this happens, the vertebral bones can fracture, leading to the formation of a hump. Symptoms associated with dowager's hump include muscle fatigue, difficulty breathing due to restriction of lung movement, chronic pain in back and shoulders, and overall stiffness.

Text Neck Causing Bone Growth in Children

Recent research reported through the *Washington Post* on June 25, 2019, and conducted by Dr. David Shahar and Mark Sayers at the University of the Sunshine Coast in Australia, has shown that texting may be to blame for younger individuals growing bone spurs on the base of their skulls. Bone spurs can be formed when repetitive motion, such as tilting the head forward, damages cartilage protecting the facet joints. This particular bone spur is typically seen when people get older and is associated with poor posture. The authors state that the forward head tilt experienced while texting or looking down "shifts weight from the spine to the muscles at the back of the head, possibly causing bone growth in the connecting tendons and ligaments." This results in a "hornlike" protuberance at the base of the skull.

Can you spot the problems associated with these texters?

Here's a hint: focus on how their posture is impacting their health.

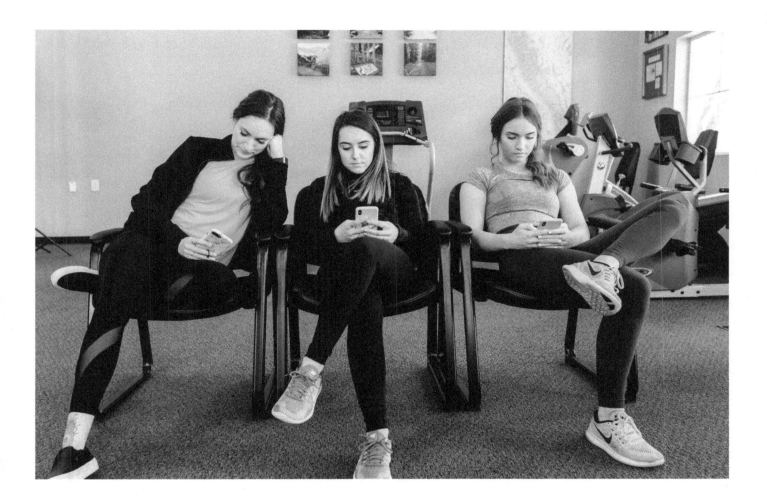

Let's Take a Look...

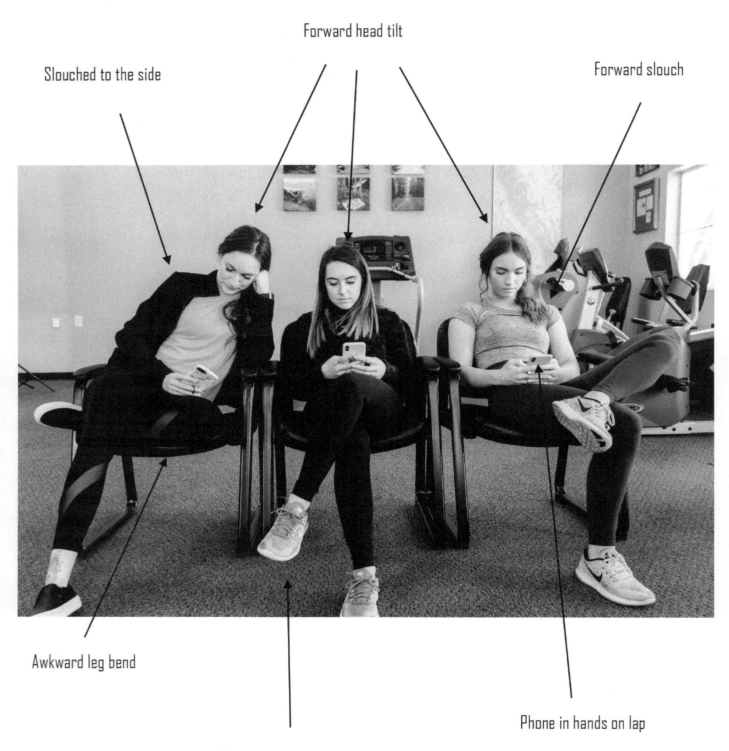

Forward head tilt

Slouched to the side

Forward slouch

Awkward leg bend

Phone in hands on lap

Feet not resting flat on the ground

A better way to text

Cervical lordosis maintained, only eyes looking down, 0-degree head tilt

Shoulders back

Arms raised (not resting in lap)

Lumbar lordosis established

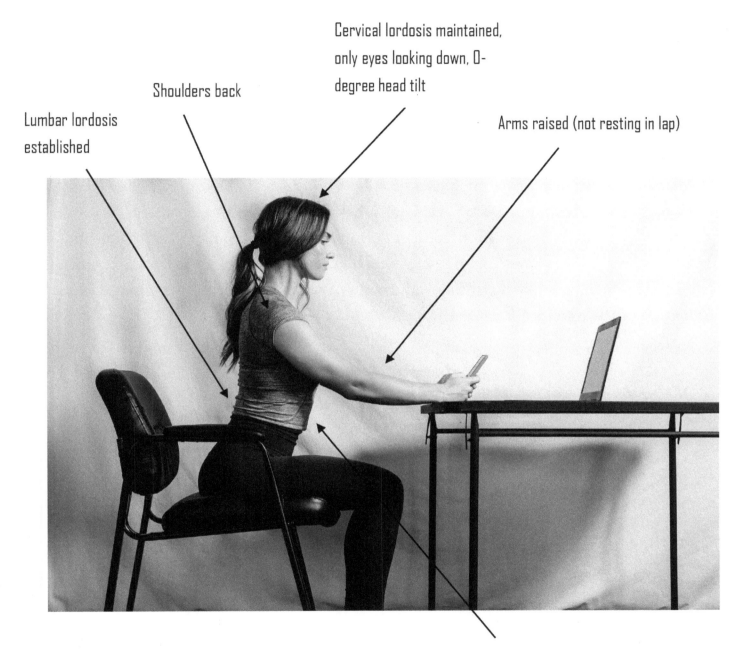

Abdominal Muscle Activation to stabilize the body and hold an upright position

Chapter 5
Sitting and Your Thoracic Spine

When the body is forced to be in a seated position for long periods of time, each region of the spine can be affected. Although many people report pain in the neck and lower back regions of the body, the thoracic spine experiences its own set of issues. The thoracic spine contributes to about "33% of functional neck movement," making it an important component of cervical mobility. Sedentary behavior through the act of sitting decreases joint and soft tissue mobility, leading to body stiffness and a high risk of pain in other areas such as the neck and arms. One study found evidence of "reduced thoracic mobility in individuals who spend more than seven hours a day sitting and get less than 150 minutes of physical activity a week." [91]

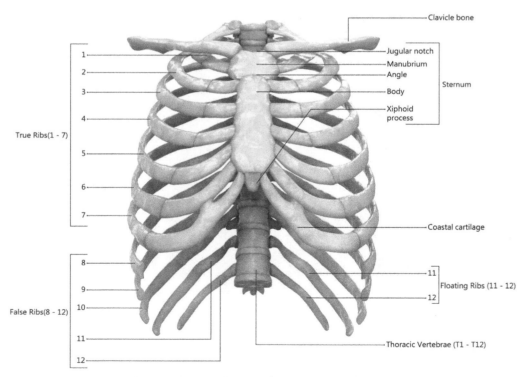

Thoracic Skeleton Anterior View

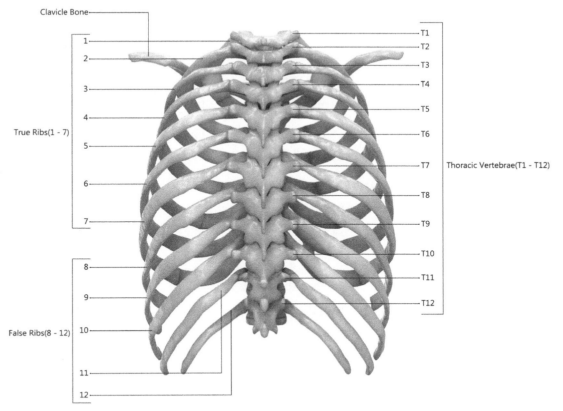

Clavicle Bone

True Ribs(1 - 7)

1
2
3
4
5
6
7

False Ribs(8 - 12)

8
9
10
11
12

T1
T2
T3
T4
T5
T6
T7
T8
T9
T10
T11
T12

Thoracic Vertebrae(T1 - T12)

Thoracic Skeleton Posterior View

Thoracic skeleton: Lateral view

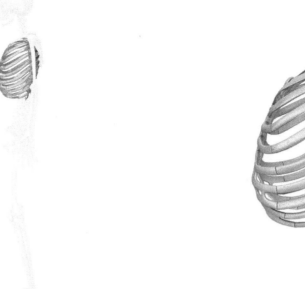

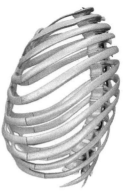

Understanding the Thoracic Region

Similar to disc problems of the cervical spine caused by sitting, the thoracic spine is also at risk. As explained in Chapter 2, the thoracic spine has a natural curve known as the kyphotic curve. When sitting for long periods of time, this curve can become exaggerated, leading to hyperkyphosis. This developed condition can become even more detrimental over time as the anterior vertebrae begin to shorten and compress, pushing the intervertebral discs posteriorly and creating risk factors for disc problems.[13] An overexaggerated kyphotic curve has even been associated with higher mortality rates. The abnormal shape of the thoracic spine in these cases not only creates strain on the discs and vertebrae, but also leads to reduced vital capacity and even pulmonary death.[13]

Along with the discs separating each vertebra in the spine, joints known as costovertebral joints and costotransverse joints also exist. These joints connect the ribs to the vertebrae and the transverse processes of the spine and allow for movement to occur by expanding the chest to make room for air to fill the lungs. These joints, in combination with the cushioned intervertebral discs between the vertebrae, make the thoracic spine an important machine that must stay well maintained in order to function properly. Injuries and bad posture are common risk factors for joint pain and may lead to more serious issues.

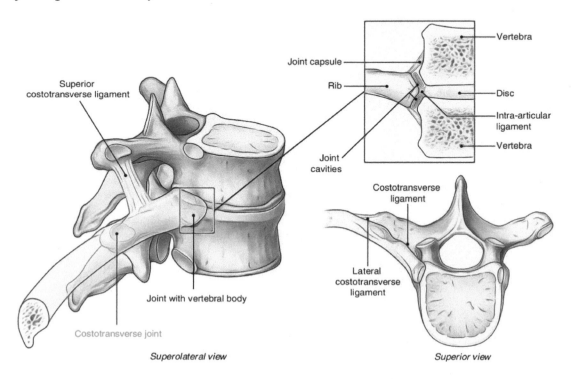

Superior costotransverse ligament

Joint capsule

Vertebra

Rib

Disc

Intra-articular ligament

Vertebra

Joint cavities

Joint with vertebral body

Costotransverse joint

Costotransverse ligament

Lateral costotransverse ligament

Superolateral view

Superior view

Breathing with Increased Kyphosis

With the sitting epidemic in full effect, all three regions of the spine are at risk. With a loss of lumbar lordosis in a seated posture comes an increased kyphotic curve in the thoracic region. The *Journal of Physical Therapy Science* explained that increased kyphosis in the thoracic spine "causes restrictions in chest expansion and respiratory muscle weakness, thereby reducing lung capacity and the thoracic cavity size and deforming vertebral column alignment."[83] When remaining in a seated position in which both the thoracic and lumbar spine have become increasingly kyphotic, the joints and tissues of the spine begin to stiffen. In order for air to flow properly in and out of the lungs, the chest must be able to easily expand fully and then relax. When the joints and tissues stiffen, breathing becomes more difficult and may limit the amount of air being brought into the lungs.

Compression Fractures

Exaggerated kyphosis can even lead to compression fractures of the vertebrae, especially when associated with any form of osteoporosis. In fact, an article published through Harvard Health Publishing states that "vertebral fractures are twice as common as hip fractures." A compression fracture involves weakening of the bone, causing it to crumble and collapse, while osteoporosis is characterized by weak, brittle bones. Therefore, a diagnosis of osteoporosis increases the chance of an individual experiencing a compression fracture of the vertebrae. Compression fractures through excessive kyphosis happen when too much pressure is placed on the front of the weakened vertebrae due to the forward leaning position of the thoracic spine, creating cracks and causing a loss of height.[102] In order to lower the risk of compression fractures of the vertebrae, it is important to maintain good, upright posture, which helps to keep pressure on the vertebrae evenly dispersed so as to not place excessive stress on the front of the vertebrae.

COMPRESSION TYPE FRACTURE OF THE VERTEBRAE

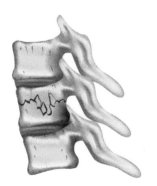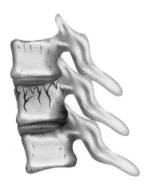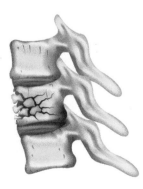

Chapter 6
Sitting and Your Lumbar Spine

Back pain is the most common cause of job-related disability and a leading contributor to missed workdays. Sitting and slouching forward produces over 185 kg of pressure on the lumbar spine and the discs between the vertebrae. Lower back pain is the leading cause of disability in people younger than 45 years old, and more than one-quarter of the working population is affected by low back pain each year.[14] Like the cervical and thoracic regions of the spine, the lumbar region may also experience damage to the vertebrae and the intervertebral discs. Chronic sitting puts individuals at an increased risk of developing lower back pain, which can be caused from either an increased or decreased lordotic curve. This chapter will offer an overview of the anatomy of the lumbar spine and the risks associated with sedentary behavior.

Common Lumbar Positions

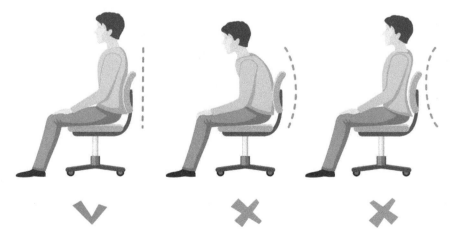

If an individual remains in a seated position for a long period of time, they may unknowingly begin to slouch, increasing the kyphotic angle, while also losing the natural lumbar curve and creating a flat back. This is shown by the middle man in the photo above.

On the other hand, an increased lordotic curve inward is referred to as hyperlordosis. Many times, if attempting to reposition the body after being seated for a while, a tendency to increase the lordotic curve in order to sit more upright arises. This can be seen in the image (previous page) with the man all the way to the right. In this position, the pelvis is tilted anteriorly, the hips are pushed back, the stomach is protruding forward, and the curve in the low back is exaggerated. Often times, this exaggerated curve is a sign of weak abdominals and tight lower back muscles. Luckily, exercises exist to combat this issue.[65]

Understanding the Lumbar Spine

In order to understand the risks associated with bad sitting posture, it is important to first recognize the anatomy of the lower back. Like the cervical and thoracic regions of the spine, the lumbar region includes its own series of joints, which consist of vertebrae, intervertebral discs, and facet joints. Although pain throughout all three regions of the back is common when sitting for hours on end, the most common area of pain reported is in the lower back. This is due to the fact that the lumbar spine supports much more of the weight of the body. While similar issues are at risk, such as disc herniation, bulge, or herniation, other problems may also emerge.

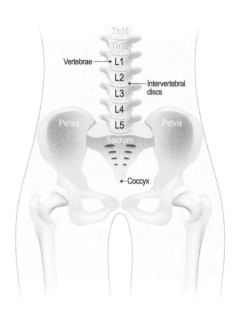

LUMBAR REGION

Discogenic Lower Back Pain

Discogenic lower back pain has been found as the most common type of lower back pain, with 39% of cases reported and about six million people living with it in the United States. An article published through the *International Journal of Biological Studies* explains that while the outer part of the discs between the vertebrae may remain undamaged, other problems, such as disc degeneration and inflammation, may internally stimulate pain receptors inside the disc. Stimulation of these receptors causes discogenic lower back pain.[66] The pain can be sharp, radiating, or even cause muscle spasms, and can be felt from the lower back to the lower legs. According to the National Spine and Pain Centers, the pain experienced by this diagnosis is typically worsened by "bending, sitting, or standing in a stationary position, and often relieved by lying down."[67]

Sciatica

In addition to disc problems that can arise from prolonged sitting, nerve problems are also a concern. The sciatic nerve, for example, is a long, thick nerve that runs from the lower back through the legs and "provides direct motor function to the hamstrings, lower extremity adductors, and indirect motor function to the calf muscles, anterior lower leg muscles, and some intrinsic foot muscles."[32] Sciatica can be worsened with flexion of the lumbar spine and twisting or bending. Irritation of this nerve can occur from intervertebral discs pushing on the nerve and creating pain that is often felt in the low back, but can also refer pain/numbness/tingling all down the leg. As previously discussed, sitting can heighten the risk of disc protrusions into the spinal cord and thus the risk of sciatic symptoms.

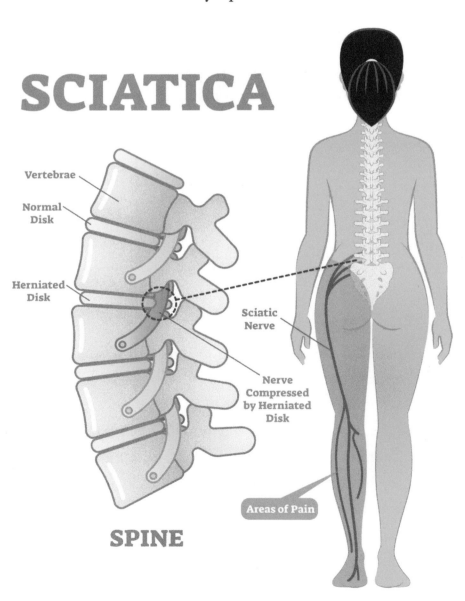

Chapter 7
Sitting and Your Hips

The hips play a major role in allowing the body to sit, which also means they are at high risk for painful symptoms and injuries. A seated position is established when the hip joint allows the femur to move forward, becoming perpendicular to the pelvis, and flexing the anterior hip muscles while extending the posterior hip muscles. The weight of much of the body then rests on the pelvis. If held for too long, this position can not only alter the normal tilt of the pelvis, but it can also create tightness and soreness around the hip region.

Anatomy of the Hips

Like the shoulders, the primary joints of the hips are referred to as ball-and-socket joints. In this case, the head of the femur acts as the "ball," and the acetabulum of the pelvic bone is the "socket." In order to support this versatile joint, muscles are constantly working to accommodate changes in position.

While sitting, the hip flexor muscles (located on the front of the hips) contract and shorten, while the hip extensor muscles (located on the back of the hips) become stretched. This can cause tightness,

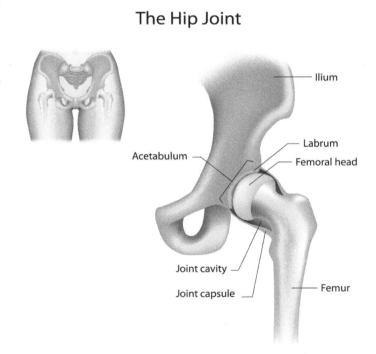

The Hip Joint

Ilium

Labrum

Acetabulum

Femoral head

Joint cavity

Joint capsule

Femur

soreness, and discomfort around the joints. If ignored, the negative effects of sitting can lead to painful problems, such as piriformis syndrome and femoroacetabular impingement.

Pelvic Tilt

Chronic sitting can lead to hip problems, such as piriformis syndrome and femoroacetabular impingement (FAI). While in a seated position, the hips are flexed, which can cause tightness and pain throughout the day. Keeping the hips in the same flexed position each day over the course of weeks, months, or even years can prove to be damaging to the joints. The problem begins with the position of the pelvis. This is because the hip joints are created from the junction of the head (top) of the femur and the acetabulum (socket) of the pelvis. The positioning of the pelvis, therefore, affects the muscles, ligaments, and tendons of the hips and can be the cause of pain. Ideally, the pelvis should be in a neutral position while sitting in order to maintain good posture and prevent painful symptoms from emerging. However, many people tend to tilt their pelvis anteriorly or posteriorly (more common) while seated. As shown in the image below, these exaggerated tilts affect the overall positioning of the spine, with an anterior tilt typically causing extension to the lumbar spine and posterior tilt causing increased flexion of the lumbar spine. With anterior pelvic tilt, the hip flexors become tight and the inward curve of the low back increases beyond normal (hyperlordosis), putting both the hips and the lumbar spine at increased risk of pain/symptoms. With posterior pelvic tilt, the abdominal muscles are weakened, as they are not being utilized to maintain an upright posture, and the normal lordotic curve is lost.

Anterior Pelvic Tilt with exaggerated lumbar lordotic surve

Posterior Pelvic Tilt with exaggerated lumbar kyphotic curve

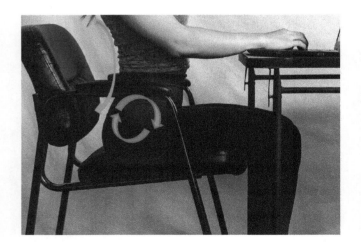

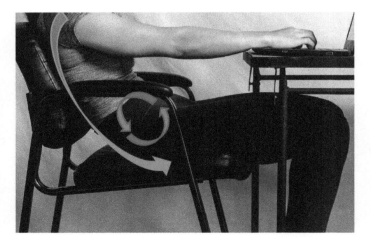

Piriformis Syndrome

The piriformis muscle plays a key role in hip external rotation. As it turns out, the sciatic nerve runs deep to this muscle, which can be compressed while sitting. If compressed, symptoms of sciatica can emerge. Conversely, if the piriformis muscle is irritated, overused, or inflamed, the sciatic nerve can flare up due to its close proximity to the muscle.

In order to avoid this issue from occurring, decrease sitting time and incorporate stretches and exercises to release tension around the sciatic nerve, and thus helping to prevent overstretching or tightening of the piriformis muscle.

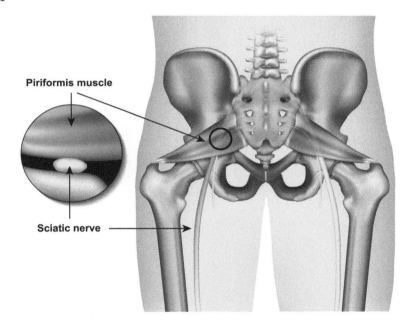

Femoroacetabular Impingement

The head of the femur sits in the acetabulum of the pelvis, creating a ball-and-socket joint to allow for movement. The acetabulum is made up of a labrum and cartilage that allows for smooth movement within the joint. When the joint is overutilized or kept in the same position, such as sitting, for an extended period of time, "conflict between the femoral neck and the edge of the acetabulum" can occur, which results in painful arthritis in the joint.[33] The resulting arthritis can lead to Femoroacetabular Impingement (FAI). There are two main types of FAI. A cam effect exists when there is a protuberance or extra bone growth off the neck or head of the femur. A pincer effect happens when extra bone extends off the acetabulum, causing impingement. When abnormalities exist on both the femoral neck and the acetabulum, the diagnosis is a mixed impingement.[33]

Chapter 8
Sitting and Your Knees

The knee joint is extremely important. It needs to be strong enough to move while holding up the weight of the body and flexible enough to allow for flexion and extension movements needed for walking, running, and other weight-bearing activities. When the body remains in a seated position for long periods of a time throughout the day, painful symptoms are likely to occur. Chronic knee pain can be caused from repetitive activities such as running and jumping, but also has the potential to develop from sitting for long periods of time.

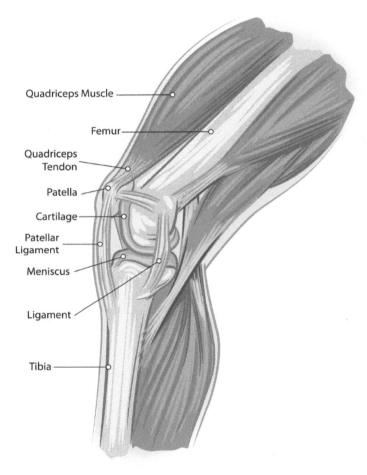

Quadriceps Muscle

Femur

Quadriceps Tendon

Patella

Cartilage

Patellar Ligament

Meniscus

Ligament

Tibia

Stiffness

Sitting with the knees in a flexed position for long periods of time can lead to intense stiffness in the joint. This can in turn make knee extension (the act of straightening the knee) more difficult and/or painful. Stiffness of a joint is characterized by reduced range of motion and flexibility. When an individual is stiff, they may experience pain, soreness, or difficulty with movement. While sitting, the quadricep muscles are in a lengthened position, while the hamstrings are in a shortened position. This stiffness is often readily apparent when watching some individuals struggle to stand up after sitting for long periods of time.

Secretary's Knee

One problem the knee is at risk of developing is a condition called patellofemoral pain syndrome, or PFPS (also known as Secretary's Knee). The Archives of Bone and Joint Surgery define PFPS as "pain surrounding the patella when sitting with bent knees for prolonged periods of time or when performing activities like ascending or descending stairs, squatting, or athletic activities."[100] When an individual is experiencing PFPS, their patella is most likely experiencing difficulty in sliding over the lower end of the femur correctly.

Patellofemoral pain syndrome can also be treated as chondromalacia patella. Chondromalacia patella is diagnosed when the cartilage under the patella has been damaged and is creating a painful, abnormal gliding of the patella over the femur. This condition can be worsened by the act of sitting and standing repetitively, causing irritation within the joint. When paired with stiffness from underused muscles while sitting, movement can be extremely painful.

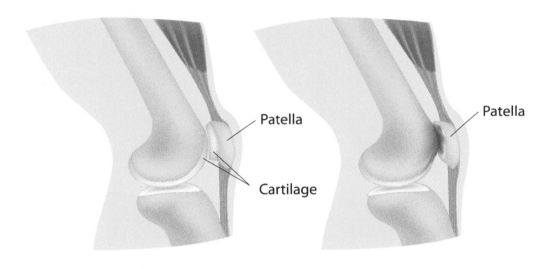

Normal   Chondromalacia

While sitting may not always be the exact cause of a pathological diagnosis it has the ability to exacerbate a problem in the joint. By keeping the knee in a bent position while sitting, the muscles surrounding the joint, such as the quadriceps, are neglected. Without strength in these supportive muscles, the joint is more prone to injury.

Chapter 9
Sitting and Your Shoulders

While sitting for long periods of time, the shoulders tend to slouch forward. This contributes to the increased flexion experienced by all three regions of the spine and the hips, causing the natural curves of the spine to be lost. Not only will the loss of the normal spinal curves potentially harm the body regions previously discussed, but it also can be extremely detrimental to the shoulders. Chronic shoulder pain can be the result of prolonged static positions (such as in sitting), or from repetitive motions, which may lead to cumulative trauma disorder, nonspecific arm pain, and shoulder impingement. Fortunately, shoulder pain can be decreased and even prevented with simple lifestyle changes that include rolling the shoulders back to reestablish posture, raising the height of the computer screen, and exercising the muscles surrounding the shoulders and upper back on a daily basis by using both stretching and strengthening techniques.

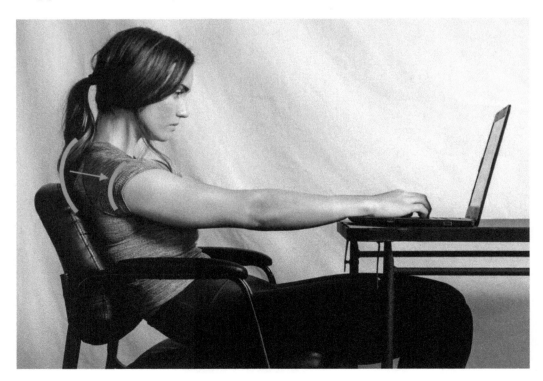

The Shoulder Joint

The shoulders are categorized as ball-and-socket joints. This means that the head of the humerus acts as a "ball," while the glenoid cavity of the scapula acts as a "socket" for the ball to fit into. In fact, this specific joint is referred to as the "glenohumeral joint" and is the main articulation of the arm to the scapula. This allows for movement such as flexion, extension, abduction, adduction, rotation, and circumduction. The glenoid labrum is located along the outside of the glenoid cavity and acts to deepen the cavity, "thereby increasing contact surface area and adding to stability."[87]

In order to protect this versatile joint, muscles, tendons, and ligaments lie all around the shoulder joint, functioning to stabilize, support, and also allow for its many different movements. Many shoulder muscles are affected by poor posture, most of which have gone through overuse, or underuse.

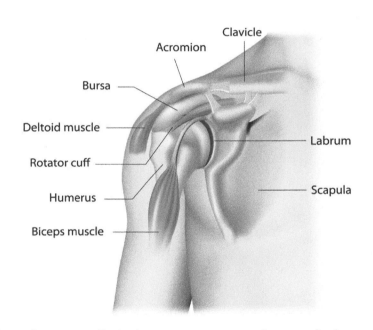

Even if the shoulder pain an individual person experiences may not be directly related to the act of sitting, the sedentary behavior leaves that person at higher risk for chronic shoulder pain and slower healing of the injured or affected areas. It is important to understand the repercussions of poor sitting posture in order to help prevent further injury to prevent further damage to the shoulder joint and promote healthy healing. Some injuries that may not be caused by sitting but may be worsened by the sedentary behavior are outlined in the rest of the chapter. While each diagnosis may be different, many can be helped with changes in posture and the combination of stretching and strengthening of the affected area.

Cumulative Trauma Disorder

Cumulative trauma disorder is characterized by pain in the area of overuse, such as the shoulders in this case. Examples of repetitive motions that affect the shoulders include moving a computer mouse around constantly, moving papers around on a desk, and using machinery. Two types of cumulative trauma disorders in the shoulder include rotator cuff tendonitis, which is the inflammation of the rotator cuff tendons in the shoulders, and bursitis. Bursitis is the result of inflammation of the bursae around the shoulder joint. Shoulder pain can also emerge from sitting if the individual has bad posture and continues to hold the same position for a prolonged period of time.[54] When this happens, the muscles in the front of the chest can become shorter and tighter.

Forward Shoulder Posture

When a person sits at a desk for long periods of time, the shoulders tend to slouch forward, following the head and rounding the upper back. When this happens, muscles and tissues of the shoulders are pulled and stretched, while muscles of the chest become tight and short. If done for prolonged periods of time without stretching and strengthening of the shoulder muscles or reestablishing good posture, pain and stiffness around the affected areas can occur.

Nonspecific Arm Pain

Nonspecific arm pain (NSAP) is also known as a repetitive strain injury and "describes the common problem of upper limb pain and functional impairment without objective physical findings."[88] It has been found that maintaining a good upper body posture protects against NSAP. This could possibly be due to the fact that postural misalignment experienced with forward shoulder posture is often associated with neuropathy of the median nerve. One study found that shoulder or scapular protraction may put the median nerve at risk because nerve movement is reduced when shoulders are slouched forward and joints change positions.[88]

Shoulder Impingement

One injury that can result from poor shoulder posture is shoulder impingement. Impingement of the shoulder is similar to FAI (Chapter Seven) in the way that something is interfering with the joint's normal functioning. In the case of the shoulder, impingement can result from a tendon, typically the rotator cuff tendons, getting caught within the subacromial space. The Mayo Clinic explains that slouched posture not only contributes to weakening muscles of the upper back and neck but also changes the positioning of the shoulder blade. When the shoulder is moved out of its normal position, space between the bones and the tendons can be compromised, leading to a higher risk of impingement.[94] The impingement can lead to inflammation of the tendons, which might be felt as pain and/or loss of range of motion in the shoulder.

Chapter 10
Sitting and Your Posture

Is it chronic sitting or poor posture while sitting that is most contributing to this unhealthy epidemic across America and much of the modernized world? We know sitting all day is detrimental to your health, but how much of the negative effects are coming from your poor sitting posture? A study published through the American Posture Institute found that people with hyperkyphotic posture, meaning extremely hunched forward, have a 144% greater rate of mortality.[38] Certain chairs, such as saddle chairs, stability ball chairs, and kneeling chairs, are aimed to improve sitting posture. If we can improve our posture but continue to sit for the length of a typical workday and more, are we less likely to suffer from the effects of sitting?

Posture, as a word on its own, is "a position in which you hold your body upright against gravity while standing, sitting, or lying down."[48] Many individuals experience static tissue loading while sitting in the same position for a long period of time. This means that pressure is loaded onto the tissues, while the body stays in one place without moving. This pressure often causes symptoms of stiffness and even soreness.

Postures can be good or bad and may be influenced not only by whether the person is sitting or standing, but also the individual person's biomechanics. In order to understand the problems associated with bad posture, we must first understand what would be considered "good" posture.

Good Posture

The Cleveland Clinic describes good posture as a position in which "the least strain is placed on supporting muscles and ligaments during movement or weight-bearing activities."[48] The article goes on to explain that when you keep the bones and joints in correct alignment, there will be less stress on the ligaments around the spine, less energy will be required to maintain the position, and the spine will be less likely to become fixed in incorrect positions. In other words, maintaining the spine's natural curves, rather than hyperextending or hypoextending the regions, will allow for proper movement and control without the symptoms of pain or soreness. The three main postural positions are seated, standing, or lying down. Each of these positions have their own do's and don'ts when it comes to proper posture.

Sitting Posture

Maintaining a correct sitting posture throughout the day can be very challenging. In order to prevent the occurrence of unpleasant symptoms associated with bad sitting posture, it is important to understand how to find and maintain a good siting posture. To have a good sitting posture, the natural curves of the spine must be maintained. In order to do this, the individual should sit up straight with the shoulders back and the butt to the back of the chair.[48] Pay attention to the lower extremities; if the feet do not touch the floor, use a footrest and do not cross the legs. The ankles should be slightly in front of the knees, and the knees should be at or below the level of the hips. If back support is available, make sure it allows for a natural lumbar curve, not overly exaggerated, but not forcing the back to be flat against the chair either. If no support is available, try using a rolled-up towel or a small pillow. Having these items will also act as a reminder to keep the back naturally arched rather than slouched. Finally, forearms should be parallel to the ground, and shoulders should be relaxed.[50]

Tips for Reestablishing Good Sitting Posture

- Put a small sticky note in the bottom corner of your computer, so that when you glance at it, it acts as a reminder to correct your posture. On the note, you can write "Posture." This is especially helpful for those who work in an office setting where sitting all day is common.

- The Cleveland Clinic suggests sitting at the end of your chair and slouching. Then, draw yourself up, exaggerating the curve of the back as much as possible, and hold the position for a few seconds. Finally, slightly release that position about 10 degrees.

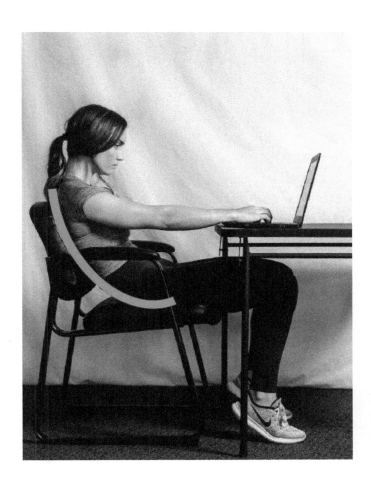
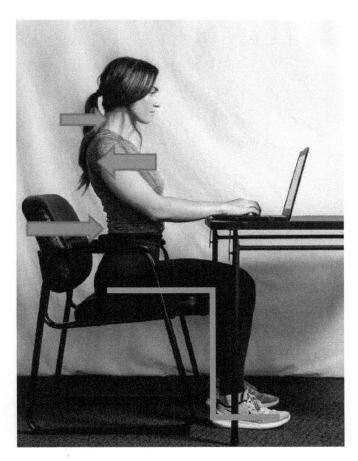

Standing Posture

Standing introduces many postural shifts that affect the shoulders, spine, and hips. This may be seen in individuals who spend much of their day on their feet. An article published through Spine Health explains that keeping the head directly over the shoulders, the shoulders directly over the pelvis, the abdominal muscles tight, and knees unlocked will assist in maintaining proper standing posture.[49] The American Chiropractic Association suggests keeping feet shoulder width apart, placing weight in the balls of the feet, and allowing the arms to hang natural at the sides of the body. If standing for long periods of time, practice weight shifting from the toes to the heels of the feet.[50]

Tips for Reestablishing Good Standing Posture

- The Harvard Medical School offers a simple tip if good standing posture is lost throughout the day by utilizing imagery. The imagery is of a straight line passing through the body, with a cord attached to the head pulling upward, as if to make the body taller.[51]

- An article published through Paleo Plan suggests visualizing the shoulders being put in your back pockets. This will put the shoulders in a more correct (posterior) position, while also forcing muscles in the back to engage.

- The article goes on to explain that standing with the upper back, butt, heels, and back of head against a wall can be beneficial in re-establishing proper standing posture.[52]

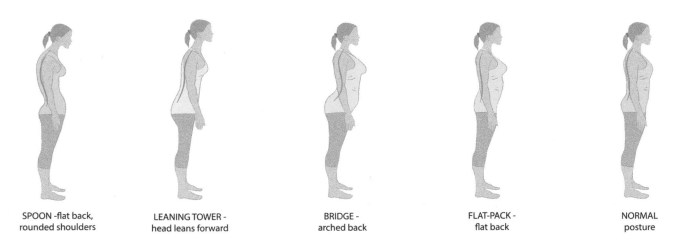

SPOON -flat back,   LEANING TOWER -   BRIDGE -   FLAT-PACK -   NORMAL
rounded shoulders   head leans forward   arched back   flat back   posture

Lying Posture

While lying down to sleep or relax, it is still just as important to maintain the natural spinal curves as it is with standing or sitting. This can often be done with the help of pillows, rather than relying on constant activation of muscles to keep a certain position. Step one to finding an adequate sleeping position is acquiring a proper mattress to not only fit the needs of your body, but also be comfortable enough to sleep in. Although firm mattresses are typically recommended, they are not always enjoyed, so it is best to go with the one that brings the most comfort. The second step to correcting posture while lying down is to place your pillow under your head, but not under the shoulders. This will allow the head to be more in line with the shoulders, rather than putting strain on the neck muscles.[48] This also means that the pillow must be at a thickness that allows for proper alignment of the head with the shoulders; pillows that are too thick or too thin will cause the head to be over- or undersupported.

The next step would be to find a comfortable sleeping position that will offer the best results for your posture. The National Sleep Foundation explains that while only 8% of people sleep on their back, it is actually the most recommended position in terms of maintaining good sleep

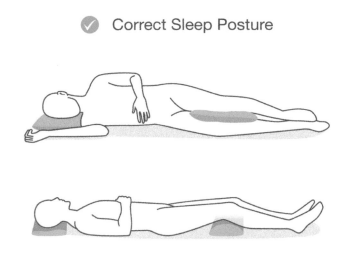

✓ Correct Sleep Posture

posture.[55] This position offers the possibility of using a pillow to support the lumbar spine and a pillow to go under the knees for optimal sleep posture.[48] A more common position is one in which the individual sleeps on their side, something 15% of adults do. The third sleep option is the fetal position, which has proven to be more popular, as 41% of adults choose this position. Although the fetal position has shown to be beneficial for pregnant women to allow for increased blood circulation throughout the body and to the fetus, it can be dangerous to those who choose this position on a nightly basis. This is because when the body is tightly curled with the torso hunched forward, the diaphragm is constricted, making breathing difficult.[55] This position can be improved by placing a pillow between the knees to lessen strain on the hips and straightening out the body. The final position, and perhaps the most detrimental to the body, is lying on the stomach. By lying on your stomach, pressure is placed on muscles, organs, and joints, leading to soreness, pain, and difficulty breathing. In addition, it is difficult to find and maintain a natural spinal curvature. If you must sleep on your stomach, try placing a pillow on your forehead, allowing the neck to line up with the shoulders while still allowing for proper airflow.

The Effects of Sitting on Walking Posture

Walking is an aspect of daily living that can be affected by prolonged sitting. As we know, sitting tightens the hip flexors by shortening the sarcomeres, so by the time it is necessary to stand, a feeling of stiffness or even soreness may encompass the body. When this happens, walking posture begins to lose shape and may even lead to painful symptoms. Tight hip flexor muscles cause the upper body to compensate by hunching forward, and arching the lower back, resulting in a flattening of the inward lumbar curve (hypolordosis). Now, not only are

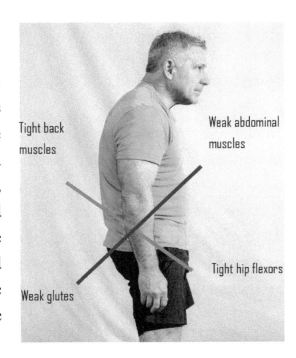

Tight back muscles

Weak abdominal muscles

Tight hip flexors

Weak glutes

the hips tight, but the entire spine also is straining to keep the body upright to allow for walking, and the knees are next in line to suffer.

Certain muscles surround the hip, allowing for movement of the leg. If these muscles become weak (from excessive siting or otherwise), the natural position of the legs while walking or sitting may be compromised and cause the leg to turn inward, putting extra stress on the knee joint. If the knee is turned inward, the ankles can also be affected by turning the feet outward, causing overpronation. Overpronation poses problems of its own, leading to flat feet and loosened joints that may cause bones to shift.[68]

Posture as We Age

Starting at around 30 years of age, our skeletal posture starts to change, resulting in changes to height, gait posture, and ability to maintain a fully upright postural position, MUSC Health explains that "on average, a person will lose about half an inch of height every 10 years from their peak height."[63] This change is due to the intervertebral discs that act as joints between the vertebrae in the spine becoming less hydrated, as explained in Chapter Four. As a "normal" side effect of aging, the discs tend to harden and lose flexibility, decreasing their ability to act as a cushioned barrier between the vertebrae. Sarcopenia, or loss of muscle mass, is another risk factor of aging. With less use, muscles will shrink and can even be replaced by fat and/ or fibrous tissue, which can further weaken the muscles. An increase in the amount of fat throughout the body can also alter the spine's ability to maintain proper posture due to the extra weight that needs to be supported. Changes in intervertebral discs, along with weakening muscles and weight redistribution, can each contribute to poor posture, typically causing the spine to stoop forward and leading to painful symptoms.[63]

In one study, groups of women 60-90 years of age were evaluated and showed gradual increases in thoracic kyphosis depth with older age. The study went on to explain that with diminishing muscle strength associated with age, elderly people will try to balance the fluctuating weight of their body by adjusting their spine, which can negatively impact posture.[64] The forward movement of the spine caused by excessive hyperkyphosis can even move the individual's center of gravity forward, affecting balance and putting the elderly person at risk for dizziness issues and an increased chance of suffering a fall.

Posture Development & Sitting Among the Younger Generation

The Heart Foundation found that children spend, on average, 7.5 hours of sitting per day on a typical Monday through Friday school week. This includes time taken to eat breakfast, ride to school, sit in class, eat lunch, ride home, do homework, and play games and/or watch television in the evening.[39] Since children are highly influenced by those around them (mainly family and friends), it is important that those role models discourage sitting time and encourage movement on a daily basis. The same article explained that "from aged two years, and possibly younger, children who watch less than an hour of television a day have a lower risk of becoming overweight" having a lower caloric energy intake and conversely eat more nutrient-rich foods than children who watch more television.[39]

Childhood growth and development can be heavily affected by their methods of upbringing, such as whether or not they spent large amounts of their day seated. Sitting has the ability to diminish academic achievement, language skills, and overall cognitive development.

Attention Spans

Dr. Mark Benden conducted a study over the course of two years in classrooms of second, third, and fourth graders, all of which added up to 282 students. He gave the students the options to either sit on a stool or stand throughout class time. He then examined the children's behaviors throughout class, such as how many times they wrote on their paper, looked at their teacher, or got distracted by peers. He concluded that those who chose to stand during class were 12-25% percent more engaged in class than those who were sitting.[40] This increase in engagement is especially relevant in today's society, with reports of attention deficit disorder and attention deficit hyperactivity disorder on the rise, both of which cause children to have a more difficult time focusing their attention.

Academic Performance

A study published in a journal called *Child Development* followed over 6,000 students for five years, starting in kindergarten, and found that children who had been considered obese during that time period scored lower math scores than those who had not been considered obese.[40] Dr. Robert Siegel believes this to be influenced by lack of physical activity, which can affect a child's "brainpower at the cellular level." In today's society, much of a child's physical activity has been replaced by activities that allow sitting. If more sitting leads to higher levels of obesity, then academic performance may also be at risk.

W Sitting

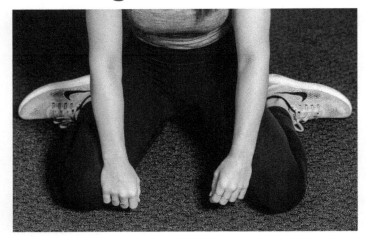

One position children commonly use while sitting on the ground is known as the *W* position. This position is characterized by the legs bent and sprawled out to the sides of the hips, as shown in the image. While many children may find this position comfortable, the strain placed on the legs proves to be detrimental to their health. North Shore Pediatric Therapy explains that sitting in this position "puts undue stress on the hip abductors, hamstrings, internal rotators, and heel cords" which can lead to more serious problems in the future, such as hip dislocation.[41] This position causes certain muscles to become tight, which can permanently shorten the muscle and "affect coordination, balance, and development of motor skills." The position allows the child to feel better supported, but simultaneously prevents them from weight shifting. Without activating the postural muscles utilized during weight shifting, the child may find it difficult to maintain stability while playing and reaching forward in any seated position.

In order to avoid possible deformities and developmental delays, other sitting positions are recommended for children. The three most common accepted sitting positions are crisscross, side sit, and long sit, all of which are shown in the images below.

Criss-Cross Side Sit Long Sit

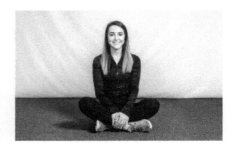
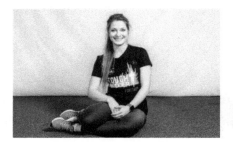
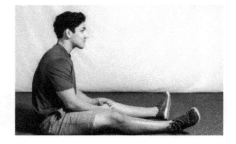

Posture, Sitting, and Developmental Concerns

Whether sitting in the *W* position, leaning over a test in class, or wearing a heavy backpack, children's postures are constantly put to the test. In a society dominated by video games, cell phones, and computers, the importance of good posture is often overlooked or even forgotten. It has been proven that there is a relationship between children who sit for long periods of time each day and their higher risk for being overweight or obese. Unfortunately, a relationship has also been shown between those who are overweight or obese and the risk factor of acquiring bad posture. A study published through the *European Journal of Pediatrics* found that in the age group between three and eighteen, the prevalence rates of those with postural problems was 69.2% and 78.6% in the overweight and obese category, respectively.[53] Elizabeth Benney, a developmental therapist, explains that when a child "w-sits, curls his toes, extends an arm, elevates his shoulder, or tucks his chin," he may be attempting to compensate for poor posture.[57]

Is It Poor Posture Or Sitting That's Killing Us?

Bad posture has proven to be detrimental to physical well-being, affecting the entire body and leading to painful symptoms. When overused, the act of sitting can be just as dangerous as simply having bad posture. The more time an individual spends in a seated position, the less time the body is utilizing important muscles, which can lead to higher health risks. However, evaluating posture while sitting versus standing is crucial in understanding the answer to the question.

A study done by the *European Spine Journal* evaluated 25 people with forward head posture (FHP) and 25 normal people. The craniovertebral angle (CVA) was measured to assess the degree of FHP each person experienced while in a seated position and while standing.[62] The CVA identifies the extent of FHP of an individual by measuring the angle between the head and the seventh cervical vertebrae. The smaller the angle, the more forward flexed the cervical spine is and the greater the FHP. The larger the CVA, the more upright or extended the head is, creating less of a FHP. The study found that the CVA was increased in sitting posture compared to standing posture.[62]

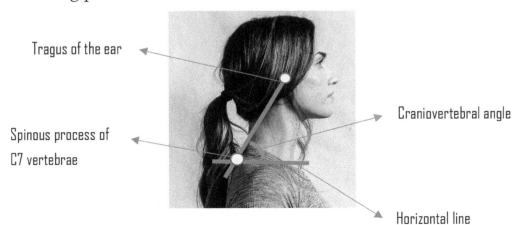

Tragus of the ear

Spinous process of
C7 vertebrae

Craniovertebral angle

Horizontal line

While posture can be influenced in different positions, while walking, and even as we age, there is much that can be done to combat the negative effects of bad posture on the body. Following proper posture guidelines, exercising to maintain muscle mass, and understanding the benefits of maintaining a stable upright position can help to lessen the risk of posture-related problems.

Postural Aids

Now that we understand the important role posture plays in our everyday lives, we can explore methods to improve postural abnormalities in the hopes of preventing further damage to the body. This section will show postural aids utilized while on the move, in one area, and even while sleeping.

"On the Move" Braces

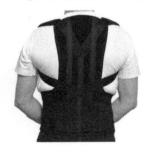

This brace wraps around the lower back, extends up the back, and wraps around the shoulders. In doing so, the shoulders are pulled back and a proper, upright position is maintained. This brace is beneficial in preventing excessive kyphosis while also providing support in the lower back. It can also provide extra support while lifting, pushing, and pulling objects.

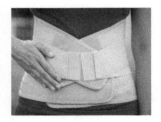

Unlike the brace mentioned above, this brace wraps around the lower back, extends up the back, and wraps around the shoulders. In doing so, the shoulders are pulled back and a proper, upright position is maintained. This brace is beneficial in preventing excessive kyphosis while also providing support in the lower back. It can also work as extra support while lifting, pushing, and pulling objects.

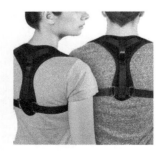

This brace focuses on the upper body. It wraps around the front of the shoulders, pulling them back and preventing forward shoulder posture. This brace can be worn while sitting, standing, or walking.

Stationary Aids

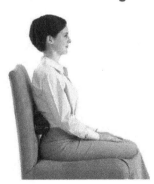

While sitting at a desk, in a car, or in front of a television, it is important to maintain proper posture in order to prevent aches and pains. Creating support for the lower back will assist in reestablishing and maintaining good spinal alignment. This can be done by placing a rolled-up towel or small pillow behind the lower back and curling the body around it. The lumbar support created by the towel/pillow will help keep the natural lordotic curve and help prevent it from flattening out.

Sleep Aids

In addition to braces that can be worn throughout the day, there are also ways to target painful problem areas while asleep. Since sleeping gives the body time to heal and rejuvenate, it is important to focus on the positioning of the head, shoulders, back, and legs. Details on the basics of proper sleeping posture were discussed earlier in this chapter.

Waking up with a kink in the neck can be frustrating, but developing chronic pain from poor sleeping posture can be life-altering. One way to assist in neck stability while sleeping is to roll up a towel or small blanket and place it under the neck while keeping the head on the pillow. This position will keep the neck from rolling forward or back and continues to work even when lying on the back or on either side. The towel or blanket mimics what some might call a "cervical roll." A study in the *Journal of Sports Medicine and Physical Fitness* found that when used correctly, the cervical roll "maintains an appropriate cervical curvature, reducing intra-disc pressure, allowing a better distribution of loads between cervical discs. The study evaluated 12 athletes who had reported chronic neck pain. Each athlete kept track of their experience with the cervical roll, and 80% reported experiencing better sleep and a relief of their neck pain. In addition, the study also stated that the pillow's shape "facilitates breathing and avoids the narrowing of the airway due to the incorrect position during the sleep."[93] One way to help prevent back pain is by placing a pillow (or two) under the knees, allowing the legs to comfortably rest on top. The pillow(s) will take pressure off the back by preventing it from arching and creating a more neutral position.

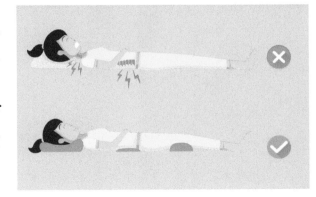

Chapter 11
Stretching While Sitting

Philosophy of Stretching

Human movement is dependent on the amount of range of motion (ROM) available in your joints. Therefore, it is important to achieve and maintain good range of motion to all your joints in order to help maintain a healthy and normal functioning musculoskeletal system. Daily stretching should be a part of every individual's overall fitness and health plan. However, the manner in which you stretch may also be important. Stretching can be classified as either static (nonmovement stretch; think three sets of 30 second holds) or dynamic (muscles and joints move to achieve the stretch; think repeated movements or stretching on and off). The good news is that stretching, whether static or dynamic, has proven to improve joint range of motion. The bad news is that static stretching has been shown to create an acute loss of muscle strength termed "stretching induced strength loss." Also, static stretching immediately prior to exercise or physical activity actually results in decreased physical performance.[103] Additionally, holding stretches for long duration can create increase strain and pain, potentially inhibiting the ability of the tissue to relax and lengthen. In contrast, dynamic stretching has been shown to improve acute muscle power as well as physical performance. I subscribe to the philosophy that "motion is lotion." You need to move your joints and muscles when stretching. This type of dynamic stretching lubricates your joints, heats up muscles, improves blood flow, and better prepares the body for physical activity. A summary of these benefits are as follows:

- Increased circulation of synovial fluid, which lubricates joints

- Increased blood flow to the joints, which helps to nourish synovial membranes

- Increased circulation of nutrients to the joints

- Activation of genes associated with cartilage repair

- Removal of cellular wastes

- Strengthening of muscles, ligaments, and tendons that provide a structure of support

Keep this dynamic stretching strategy in mind as you begin these stretching exercises. It will help if you think of "stretch on" as you move into the stretch, and then "stretch off" as you move back to the starting position. The analogy I use is to think of stretching in terms of repetitions performed like in weight training. My daily recommendations for these stretches are two sets of twelve, twice a day. For example, do twelve repetitions of the stretch, rest for a minute or two, and then do twelve more repetitions of the same stretch. Then repeat again later in the day. If that it is too much, then another strategy would be to break up your routine into upper body stretches one day and lower body stretches the next day.

Cervical Spine Retraction

Starting position: Sit with good posture and head and neck in neutral resting position. Use your hand to grab your chin between your thumb and index finger.

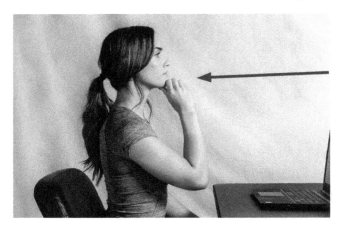

The movement: Simultaneously activate your neck muscles and push with your hand to retract your neck (push your chin straight back toward your neck). Hold the end stretch position for two or three seconds, and then release and let your neck and chin return to resting position.

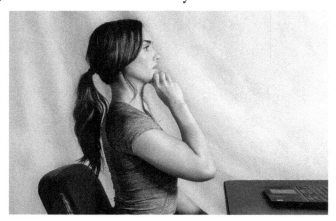

Common mistakes:

- Holding the stretch for too long
- Performing the stretch too fast (each stretch or repetition should take five to seven seconds)
- Performing too shallow of a stretch (need to push the stretch far enough to feel tension in the neck muscles at the end stretch position)
- Pushing the chin up or down while performing the stretch
- Moving your torso forward or backward during the stretch (torso should remain still and stable)
- Resisting the push of your head with your neck muscles. Relax your neck so that you get a good movement of your neck when you push your chin back toward your neck

Cervical Spine Extension

Starting position: Sit with good posture and head and neck in neutral resting position. Use your hand to grab your chin between your thumb and index finger.

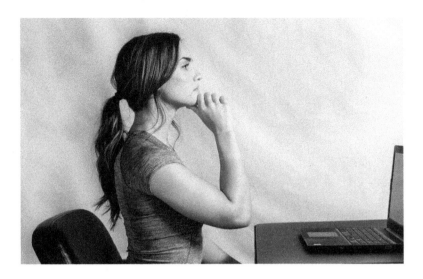

The movement: Look upward and tilt your head back so that your chin moves upward toward the ceiling. As your chin moves upward, use your thumb to apply pressure from under the chin to push it farther and farther upward toward the ceiling. Hold the end stretch position for two to three seconds, and then slowly return to the starting position.

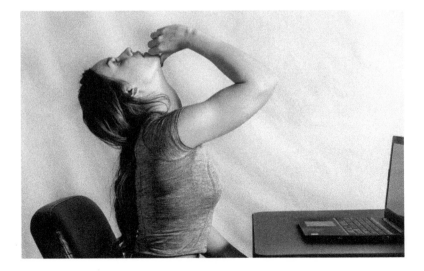

Common mistakes:
- Moving your torso as you push your chin up
- Not pushing stretch far enough (should feel tension in the neck and muscles at the end stretch position)

Thoracic Spine Extension

Starting position: Sit with good posture and your back fully against your chair (ideally three-quarters high back). Grab both of your elbows with the opposite hands.

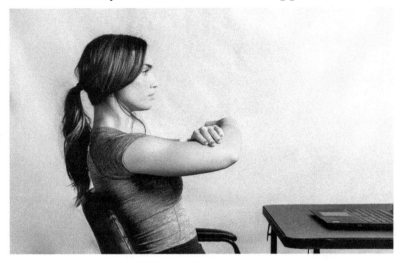

The movement: Lift your elbows toward the ceiling, and tilt your upper back over the chair. Lift your chin upward as you perform the movement. Hold the end stretch position for two to three seconds, and then slowly return to the starting position.

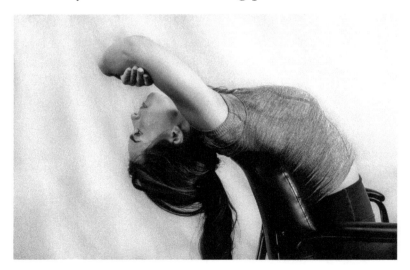

Alternative movement position: If you experience any neck strain or pain during the movement, you may try the stretch with your hands supporting the neck during the movement.

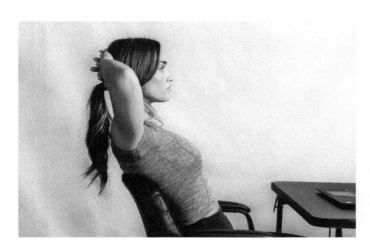
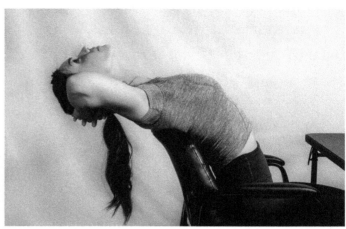

Common mistakes:

- Using a chair that is too high or too low; the top of the chair should be around the mid-scapula area (bra line for females)
- Not lifting your elbows up high enough during the movement
- Not tilting your chin up toward the ceiling during the movement

Standing Lumbar Extension

Starting position: Stand tall, turn around, and lean your hips up against a chair, counter, or couch. Place your hands down at your side, holding onto the chair for support and balance.

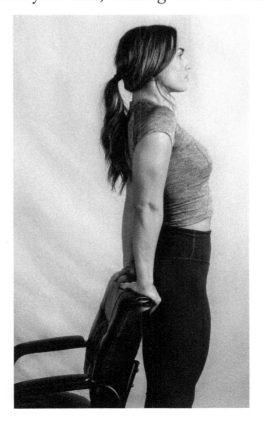

The movement: Lean backward and pivot over your chair; use your arms to stabilize and balance yourself as you lean over backward. Hold the end stretch position for two to three seconds, and then slowly return to the starting position.

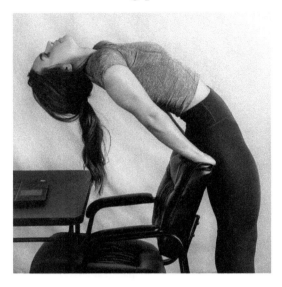

Common mistakes:

- Lifting your heels off the ground (feet should remain flat on the ground throughout the movement.)
- Not using your hands to help with balance and support during the movement
- Using too high or too low of a chair, counter, or sofa (should touch at the upper area of your backside or lower area of your low back)

Slouch/Overcorrect

Starting position: Sit with good posture and with your hands relaxed.

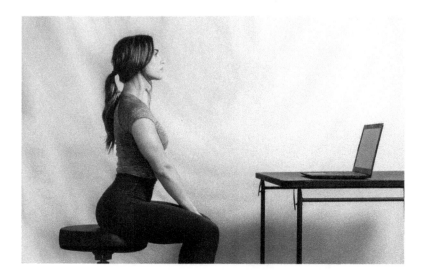

The movement: Slowly roll your hips posteriorly (backward) until you reach an end or stopping position (the slouch). Hold for a second or two, and then roll your hips anteriorly (forward) until you reach a stopping position (the overcorrect). You may place your hands over your hips to feel (and facilitate) the hips rolling forward and backward.

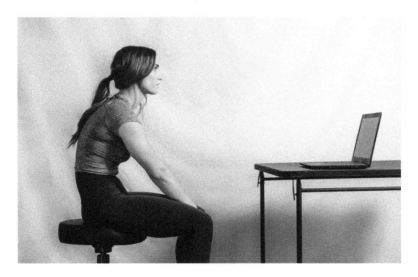

Common mistakes:
- Moving your torso forward and back (instead of letting the hips roll forward and back)
- Not rolling the hips completely forward, backward, or both

Shoulder Extension

Starting position: Kneel on one or both knees while placing both arms behind you with your hands (palms down) on top of your desk while keeping your elbow straight.

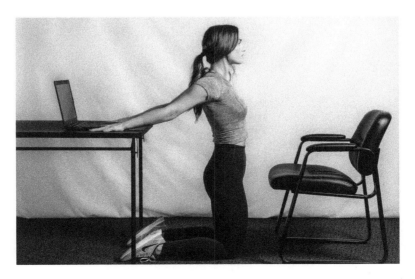

The movement: Lean slightly forward, keeping your arms on the desk, and lower your hips toward the floor by bending your knees. Hold the end stretch position for two to three seconds, and then return to the starting position.

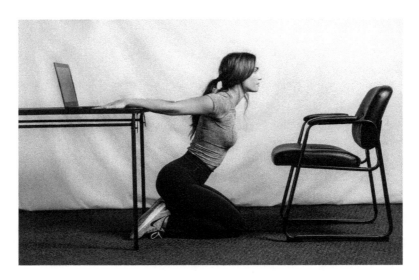

Common mistakes:
- Bending your elbows during the stretch
- Only leaning body forward instead of lowering hips toward the floor

Shoulder Internal Rotation

Starting position: While sitting, place a hand towel over your shoulder so that it is behind your back. Reach behind your back with your other arm and grab the bottom of the towel. The arm holding the bottom of the towel will be the one getting the shoulder internal rotation stretch.

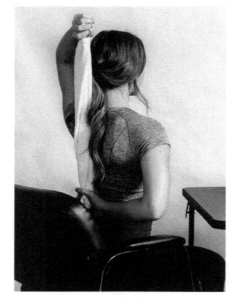

The movement: Pull the towel upward toward the ceiling with the arm holding the top of the towel. Relax the arm holding the bottom of the towel, and let it slide upward (moving up your back). Hold the end stretch position for two to three seconds, and then return to the starting position.

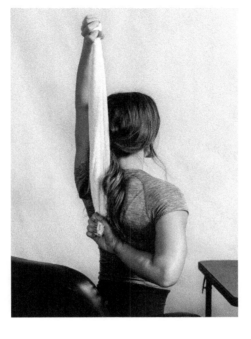

Common mistakes:
- Pulling arm horizontal versus vertical on the stretch
- Bending torso forward as you stretch the arm upward

Hip Extension (Stool)

Starting position: Place your stool behind a stable object (chair, desk, etc.). Place the front part of your lower leg on the stool. Assume good, full, upright posture.

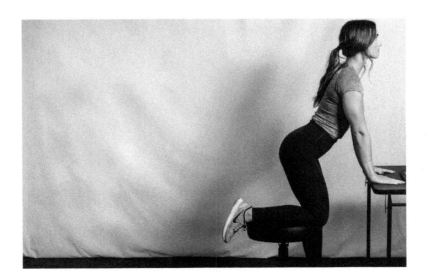

The movement: Keep your torso fully upright as you use your back leg (leg on stool) to push the stool backward behind you. Hold the end stretch position for two to three seconds, and then return to the starting position.

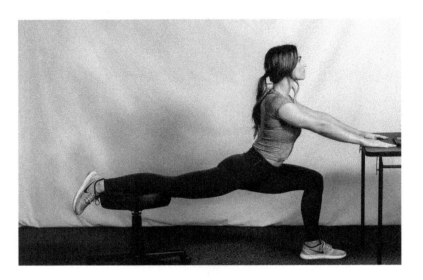

Common mistakes:
- Bending your torso forward as you perform the stretch
- Not using proper support from each side (desk/chair/etc.) as you perform the stretch

Hip Extension (Floor)

May be utilized if you don't have a stool or don't feel comfortable or safe using a stool.

Starting position: Kneel down on one knee (the target hip being stretched into extension), and bring the opposite leg forward with your front heel flat on the floor. Hold onto your desk or chair for balance/stability to better perform the stretch.

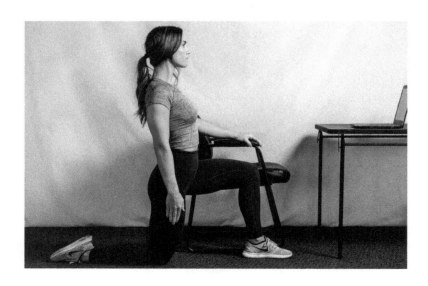

The movement: Keep your torso nice and straight (keep fully upright) as you move your front knee in a forward direction. Hold the end stretch position for two to three seconds, and then return to the starting position.

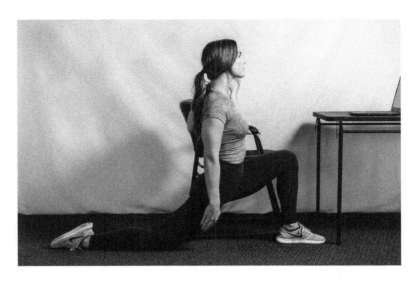

Common mistakes:
- Not having forward leg out far enough in front of you
- Leaning your torso forward as you perform the stretch
- Not having a stable object (chair/desk/etc.) to help perform the stretch fluidly and correctly

Hip Internal Rotation (Stool)

Starting position: Using your desk or a chair to balance and stabilize, stand upright with your knee or lower leg resting easily on the stool.

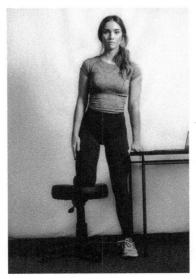

The movement: Keep your good upright posture, and turn your knee (on the stool) inward toward the midline of your body. Hold the end stretch position for two to three seconds, and then return to the starting position.

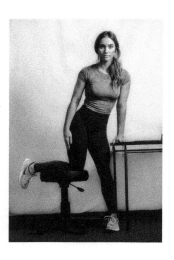

Common mistakes:
- Bending your torso forward during the stretch
- Putting too much of your body weight onto the stool during the stretch (knee/lower leg should rest easily on the stool)
- Twisting your torso outward instead of hip inward

Knee Extension

Starting position: Sit at the edge of your chair, and extend your knee straight. Lean forward over your straightened knee, and place your hands over your lower thigh (above the knee joint). Your hands should be pancaked over each other.

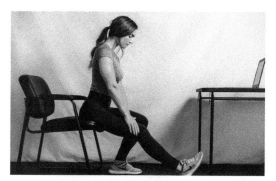

The movement: Lean slightly farther forward and use your arms and hands to push your lower thigh downward toward the floor, stretching the knee into further extension. Hold the end stretch position for two to three seconds, and then return to the starting position.

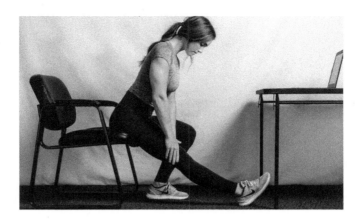

Common mistakes:

- Pushing on the knee joint itself (instead of your thigh)
- Pushing toward your feet instead of pushing down toward the floor
- Not leaning torso forward enough to get your body weight over your arms/hands

Hip External Rotation (Figure Four Stretch)

Starting Position: Sit on the edge of your chair and cross your right ankle over your left knee. Use your left hand to hold (stabilize) your right ankle still. Note: If this position is too challenging or painful, you can modify the starting position by simply placing your right foot on top of your left foot.

The movement: Use your right hand to push your right knee downward and outward until you feel a good stretch. Hold the stretch for 0 to three seconds and then return to the starting position. Repeat the exercise on the opposite leg.

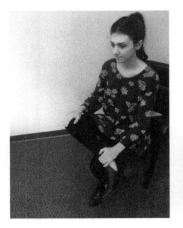 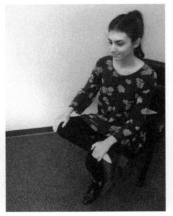 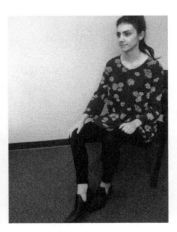 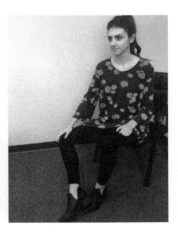

Common mistakes:

- Allowing the ankle to slide around on the knee during the stretch
- Not sitting at the edge of the chair during the stretch

Chapter 12
Good Body Mechanics

In order to understand and reduce the negative symptoms associated with bad posture, chronic sitting, and a sedentary lifestyle, it is important to learn proper techniques of movement. The term "body mechanics" involves the way humans move, such as while sitting, standing, lying down, and going about activities of daily living. It is "a term that indicates a coordinated effort of the musculoskeletal and nervous systems to maintain balance, posture, and body alignment in daily life, which is directly related to effective bodily functioning."[69] Basic principles of body mechanics include utilizing a wide base of support, keeping the back straight, and incorporating larger muscle groups when lifting in order to reduce the risk of injury.[70] This chapter will utilize the principles of body mechanics to explain proper pushing, pulling, and lifting techniques. Simply changing the way the body is positioned and the muscle groups that are activated while moving heavy objects or even picking something lightweight off the floor can lower the risk of injury and introduce new strengthening exercises.

An Overview of a Common Practice

For many people, work is a common place for incorporating body mechanics, such as when moving objects from one place to another. Unfortunately, this means that many injuries are likely to occur in jobs that require this type of movement constantly. Injuries range from simple back, neck, and shoulder problems to even more serious accidents. Ohio State University's Spine Research Institute stated that "the average cost of a back injury related workers comp claim can be $40,000 to $80,000 per employee."[89] These work-related accidents led to the creation of the Occupational Safety and Health Administration, also known as OSHA, in 1971. With OSHA, certain guidelines have been put in place to ensure safer working conditions while also providing proper training and education to employees in order to help prevent injury from occurring at the workplace.

In addition to injury at the workplace being a concern, outside activities such as heavy lifting at the gym, moving from one house to another, and even normal activities of daily living can also pose risks. Many times, a simple lesson on proper lifting, pushing, and pulling mechanics is all that is necessary to lower the risk of injury. The next few pages will outline these common practices and offer safer ways to complete these types of tasks.

Lifting An Object

- Directly face the object to be lifted and get as close to it as possible.

- Keep the elbows and arms close to the body.

- While lifting, the legs should take on the majority of the load, rather than the back. In order to do this, squat down rather than bend over. Keep a wide base of support to prepare for the load by making sure the feet are at least shoulder width apart. Proper form is achieved by maintaining a straight back, tightening the stomach muscles, bending at the knees, and looking ahead.

- Get a good handle on the object. Leaning back slightly to maintain balance can be helpful.

- Take a deep breath and exhale as you carefully stand up utilizing the muscles in the legs, and avoid twisting during the lift. To help avoid twisting, shift your feet to turn rather than your back.[79]

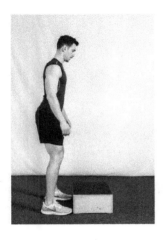 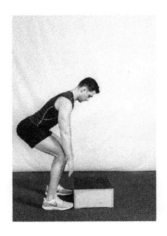 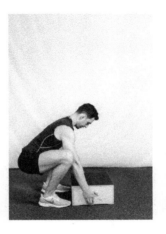 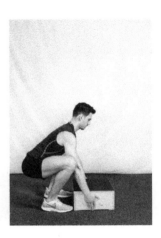

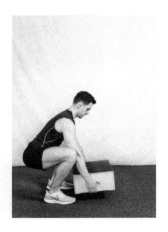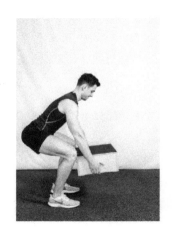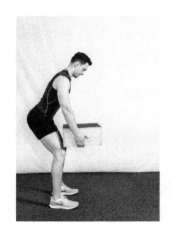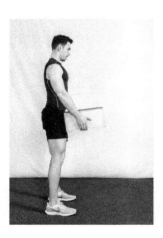

Lifting Lighter Objects

Lifting not only pertains to heavy objects; a person can still be injured while picking up something lightweight, such as a golf ball. In fact, there is a method some golfers may use, known as the "golfer's lift," that helps to protect the lower back from undo stress/strain incurred when bending down to the floor. This method can be accomplished by leaning forward, keeping one leg straight on the ground, and lifting the other leg straight back to act as a counterbalance. From here, the individual reaches out an arm to pick up the golf ball or other light object. This lift is similar to that of a single leg deadlift. The muscles predominantly utilized in this maneuver include the hamstrings, glutes, and stabilizing muscles in the back.

Golfer's Lift

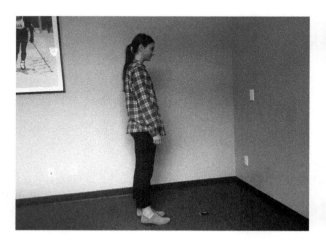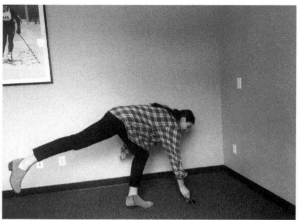

Bad Lifting

It has been found that lifting with a rounded (kyphotic) back raises pressure in the discs of the spine to an excessively high level when compared to lifting with a lordotic curve present.[79] Increasing pressure in the discs can lead to problems such as disc bulging and disc herniation.

Lifting with a rounded back also increases the risk for muscle strains, which happens when the demands placed on the muscles are too high, creating little tears. This can lead to pain, soreness, and discomfort.[80]

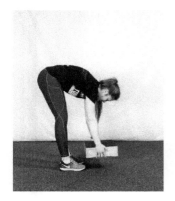 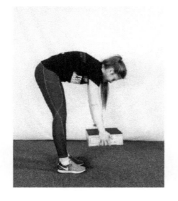 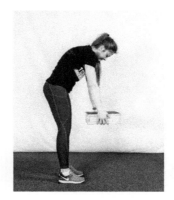 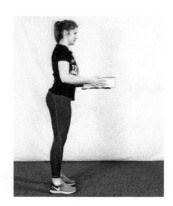

Carrying

- Your hips, shoulders, toes, and knees should stay facing the same direction.

- Keep the object close to the body.

- Avoid allowing the back to hunch forward or curve backward. If feeling fatigued, set the object down before proceeding.

DO

DON'T

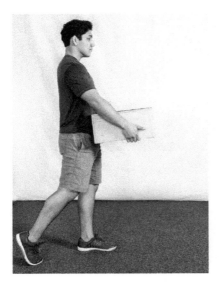 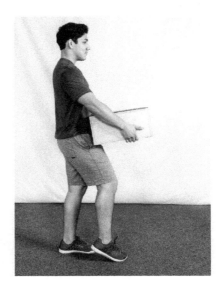

Setting The Object Down

- Think about setting the object down the same way you picked it up, but in reverse.

- Bend at the knees, not the hips. This will maintain power in the legs rather than placing unnecessary strain on the back.

- Keep the head up and the abdominals tight.

- Refrain from twisting or bending at the back. Move downward in a straight line.

- Keep the object close to the body.

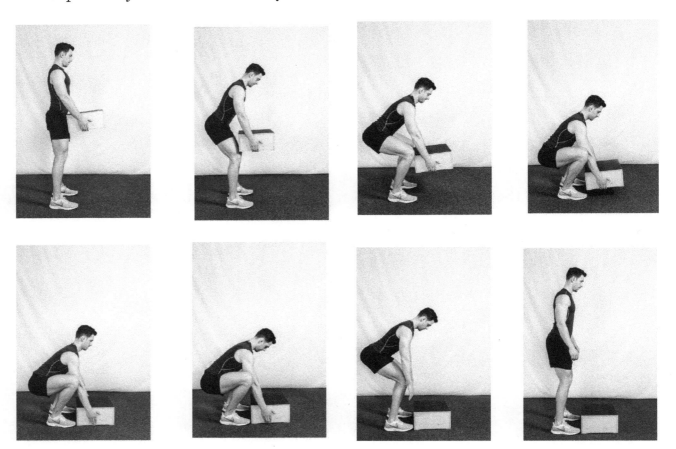

Pushing: Do's[72]

- Keeping the body in proper alignment is the first important step before attempting to push an object. This means making sure the ears, shoulders, and hips are all lined up.

Hunching the back forward or even curving it inward can put strain on the supporting back muscles and cause them to weaken while also placing overbearing load on the vertebrae.[73]

- Tighten the abdominal muscles. This will stabilize the front of the spine.

- Lean into the object, and use the legs and the force of the body to move the object forward. Focus on making the muscles in the legs work, rather than the back.

- Take small steps.

Another tip when completing pushing tasks is to increase friction between the feet and the ground in order to move the object with less effort and strain on the muscles. Slip-resistant shoes or those with extra traction are beneficial in these instances.[74]

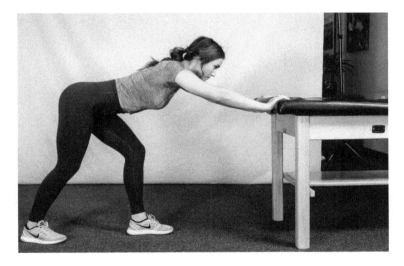

Pulling Do's
- Do face the object.
- Do bend the knees and slowly walk backward, avoiding twisting motions.
- Do put one hand on the hip if pulling with the other hand to maintain stability.
- Do lean back while keeping the spine straight and the shoulders back to allow the whole body, rather than just the back, to pull the load.

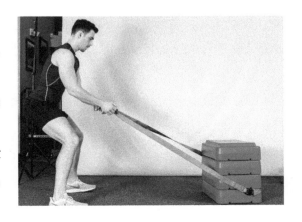

Pulling Dont's

- Do not face in the direction of travel. Facing away from the object and pulling it from behind causes the arms to be stretched and strained, forcing the shoulders and back to be put in a mechanically awkward posture.[74]
- Do not hunch the back forward or arch it backward (as shown in the image to the right). This will cause the back to take on the load of the object and can cause the muscles to become strained.

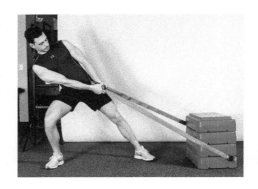

Pushing versus pulling: What to Choose

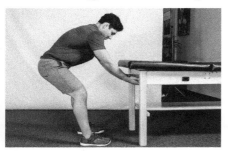

When it comes to moving heavy objects, there are certain body mechanics that must be maintained in order to ensure safety and help avoid injury. *Whenever possible, it is recommended to push objects rather than pull.* The explanation to this statement introduces a bit of physics: Isaac Newton's second law of motion states that the net force applied to an object is equal to the size of the object (mass) multiplied by its movement speed (acceleration). In other words, "when you are trying to move an object, you'll have to exert the same force whether you push or pull."[71] Although the same amount of force is exerted when pushing or pulling objects, the body moves differently depending on the motion, meaning certain muscles and joints may be working harder than others. The friction acting on an object also plays a role when determining the benefits of pushing or pulling an object.

One study was conducted with the assistance of ten women and ten men to assess spine loading throughout the lumbar spine. Participants pushed and pulled loads at three different handle heights and three different load magnitudes. The results showed that pulling loads equivalent to 30% of the individual's body weight and pushing loads at 20% would be within the margin of safety and prove to be nonproblematic.[76] In addition, the study found that after examining three different handle heights, the lowest height proved to place less stress on the spine than the middle or highest levels.

Simply put, pulling increases stress and strain on the lumbar spine muscles, while pushing is achieved through the help of the quadriceps, glutes, and hamstring muscles.

Chapter 13

Strategies for Good Spinal Health

Changes in your daily routine may be all it takes to improve your spinal health. While these changes may be small, they can make a lasting impact on the way your spine functions and handles the stresses of everyday life. Incorporating any one of these strategies may be the answer to alleviating your neck, back, or leg pain. If the strategies you choose to try seem daunting, try creating goals that you can work toward, such as trying them every other day or for intervals of time. This will make the transition easier. Now, let's look into those strategies.

Use Standing Desks

A study conducted through the Centers for Disease Control over a seven-week period found that having a desk with the ability to be raised up, allowing the person to stand while working, reduced sitting time and projected strong health benefits to those who participated. Nonsitting time was increased, which resulted in a reduction of upper back and neck pain while also improving mood states.[2] In fact, about 60% of full-time employees admit they would be more productive if they had the option to work seated or standing.[9]

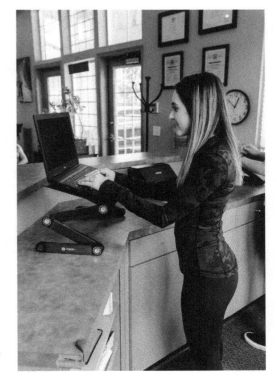

Walk or Bike to Destinations

Driving is a large contributor to the sitting epidemic. When attempting to minimize symptoms created by sitting, one might try replacing the car with walking shoes. This will save you money on gas, help the environment, and get you moving. A study conducted through the medical journal BMJ evaluated those who walk or bike to work versus those who drive. The study found that those who walk to and from work were 36% less likely to die from heart problems, and 90% of those who chose to bicycle to work met their recommended physical activity guidelines.[81] A goal of 10,000 steps may be a good motivation to walk more and sit less. Personally, I have found the Fitbit to be highly motivating to move, as I have often found myself walking around my house into the night to reach my daily goal of 20,000 steps. A variety of Fitbits are available that count daily steps and to help in motivation to walk more and sit less.

Take Standing/Walking Breaks

If the thought of walking or standing throughout the day seems daunting, try incorporating breaks of 10, 20, or 30 minutes at a time. This may include taking a walk around the block at home or standing for a period of time at work. One idea would be to go for a walk during the lunch hour and setting a phone alarm to go off every so often for a standing break. While this may not seem like much, a new study published through the Journal of the American Heart Association found "evidence that sporadic and bouted moderate-to-vigorous physical activity (MVPA) is associated with substantially reduced mortality."[90] In other words, accumulating walking bouts of ten minutes or longer has proven to be beneficial in maintaining a healthy lifestyle. My general rule is that you should not sit for more than 30 minutes straight before either taking a standing break or short walk.

Face Time

When working in an office setting, try incorporating some face to face interaction. Instead of calling another person in the office or sending an instant message, walk over to them. This will get you moving, allowing you to stretch the joints and help prevent stiffness from occur-

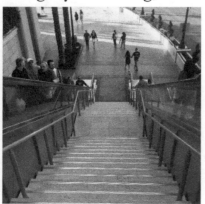

ring. In addition, it may contribute to a more interactive work environment.

Skip Elevators and Take the Stairs

If your office has multiple levels, taking the stairs can be a great way to incorporate movement into your daily routine. In fact, "climbing just eight flights of stairs a day lowers the average early mortality risk by 33%" and "just two minutes of extra stair climbing a day is enough to stop average middle age weight gain."[82]

Use a Stability/Exercise Ball as a Chair

Sitting on a stability ball can improve balance, posture, and abdominal strength while also allowing for movement to occur. This movement contributes to adequate blood flow throughout the body and may prevent muscles and ligaments from becoming tight. While on the ball, muscles in the core and throughout the length of the back are constantly working to maintain an upright posture. It can also be used during an exercise break to encourage movement throughout the day. The images below show examples of ways to sit and move on the exercise ball.

Good upright posture   Forward and back

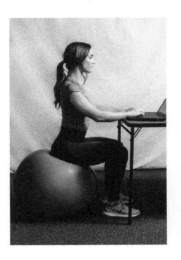 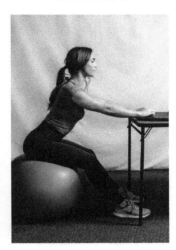

Side to side movements

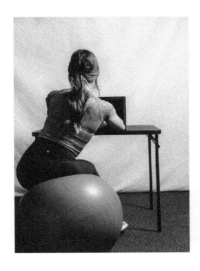 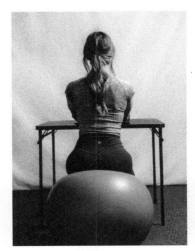 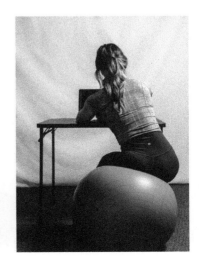

Activate Your Transverse Abdominis

The transverse abdominis is the deepest of the abdominal muscles, and is located beneath the rectus abdominis and spans across the abdomen horizontally. This muscle mimics a back-support belt in the way that it wraps around from the front of the trunk to the back, and resists lumbar flexion (it helps keep you upright). Not only does this muscle create tremendous postural support when activated, it also contains and supports organs located within the trunk. In addition, the transverse abdominis muscle may be contracted while breathing during exhalation to increase pressure in the lungs and aid in exhalation.[98] This muscle works with the pelvic floor muscles to provide stability to the lower back and pelvis. The phrase "work your core" is often heard, but what does it really mean? The transverse abdominis is a key muscle to think of when focusing on the "core." Prior to almost any movement, the transverse abdominis is activated to stabilize the low back and pelvis.

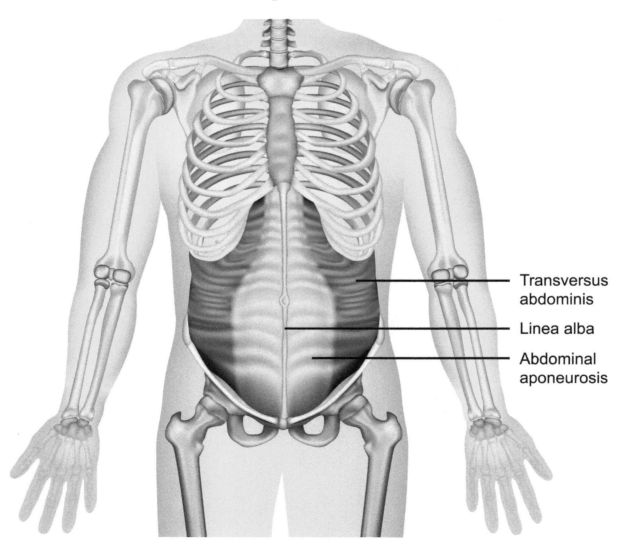

Transversus
abdominis

Linea alba

Abdominal
aponeurosis

Activation of Transverse Abdominis

Starting Position: Sit comfortably in upright position and place a finger over your belly button

Activation of Transversus Abdominis: Keep your finger still, and remove your belly button from your finger by drawing your naval inward towards your spine (think of hallowing your abdominal area)

Common Mistakes:

• Pulling your finger away from your belly button instead of the belly button away from your finger

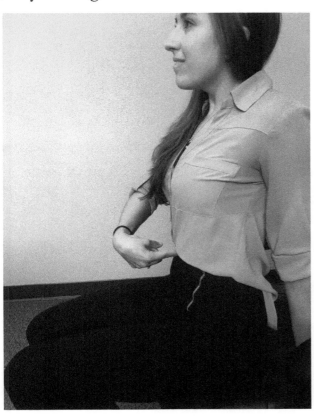 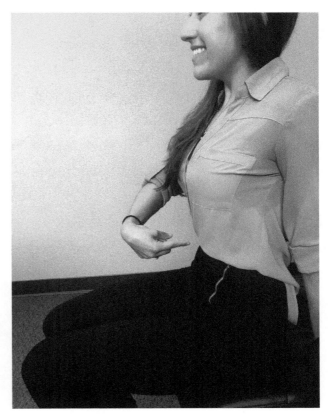

Daily Spine Stretching/Range of Motion Exercises

As I often tell my patients, stiffness is the enemy of our musculoskeletal system. Stretching of your spine (cervical/thoracic/lumbar) is vital in the prevention of spinal stiffness. Performing daily range of motion exercises will not only do wonders for your spinal health, they can help reduce stiffness throughout your body that develops from chronic sitting. The next chapter explains in detail several daily stretches that are recommended not only for the spine, but for other major joints of the body as well.

Chapter 14

Stretching to Improve Everyday Living

Stretching and strengthening weak or overused muscles is an excellent way to combat the negative effects (pain/stiffness/soreness) associated with sitting, poor posture, and overall sedentary behavior. Stretching can be done to reduce (and hopefully also prevent) injury from occurring. The exercises in this chapter are stretches that can be done as needed to help prevent or relieve pain and stiffness from affected areas. Unlike the stretches outlined in chapter 11, these may be done on any flat surface, such as the floor, and target muscles of the whole body. As noted in chapter 11, these stretches should not be performed if pain or discomfort occurs.

Lumbar Spine Rotation

Starting position: Lie on the floor/bed/yoga mat with both knees bent comfortably.

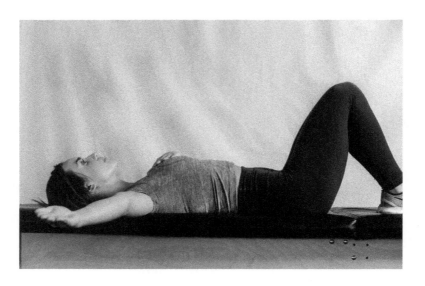

The movement: Keep both your shoulders flat. Swivel both knees to the left, hold for a couple of seconds, and then swivel both knees to the right, and hold for a couple of seconds. Let your hips roll back and forth with the movement.

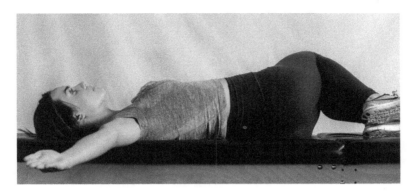

Common mistakes:
- Not keeping your knees together
- Not keeping both shoulders flat
- Not letting your hips roll back and forth with the movement

Knee Flexion (Standing)

Starting position: Stand fully upright holding onto chair, table, or other object for balance and stability. Bend your knee, and use your same-side hand to grab your foot/ankle.

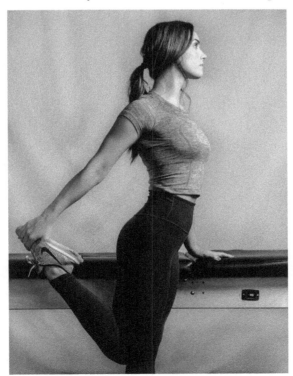

The movement: Keeping a fully upright posture, pull your ankle/foot upward and toward your buttocks region. Hold the end stretch position for a couple of seconds, and then return to the starting position. Your knee should remain pointed down toward the floor during the entire stretch.

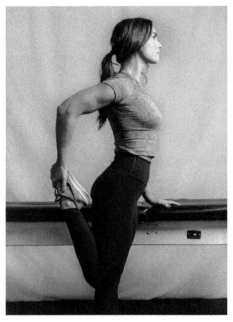

Common mistakes:
- Leaning forward as you stretch your knee
- Pulling leg forward or backward during the stretch

Knee Flexion (Quadruped Position)
Can be used if the standing knee flexion stretch is too difficult or painful to perform.
Starting position: Kneel down on both knees, and lean forward so your hands are on the floor and shoulders are over your hands.

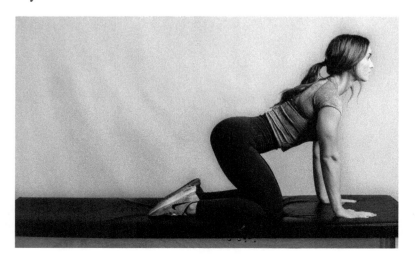

The movement: Bend your knees by leaning your hips backward so that your hips move toward your ankles. Hold the end stretch position a couple of seconds, and then return to the starting position.

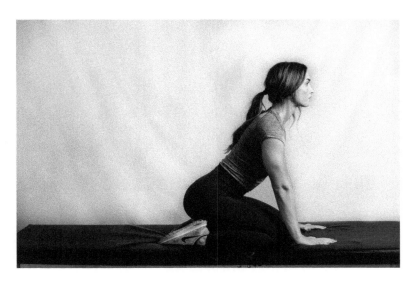

Common mistakes:
- Moving body forward instead of backward

Hip Flexion

Starting position: Lie on your back with one knee bent and one knee straight.

The movement: Reach out with both arms and grab your bent knee (may grab the front of the knee or underneath the knee). Pull your knee toward your chest, hold the end stretch a couple of seconds, and then return to the starting position.

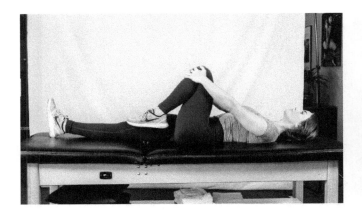
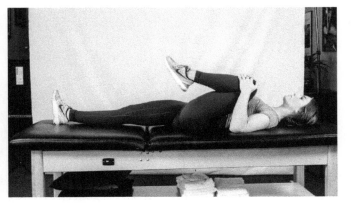

Supported: If grabbing your knee is too difficult or painful, you can wrap a towel under the knee that will be lifted. Grab each end of the towel with your hands and pull to bring the knee up.

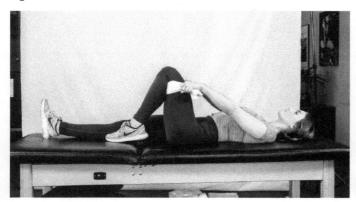 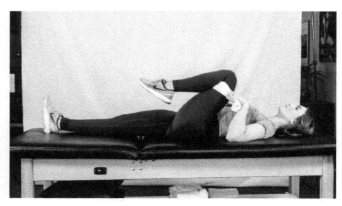

Common mistakes:
- Bending or straightening your knee during the stretch
- Pulling leg outward instead of straight toward the chest
- Not keeping your opposite knee straight during the stretch

Lumbar Flexion (Sitting)

Starting position: Sit on the edge of your chair with your legs well apart from each other.

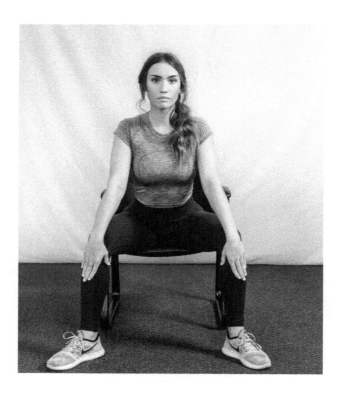

The movement: Lean your torso downward, and reach your arms toward your ankles/feet. Hold the end stretch position a couple of seconds, and then return to starting position. If you do not feel a sufficient stretch, you may grab your ankles and use your arms to pull your torso farther toward the floor for a more forceful stretch.

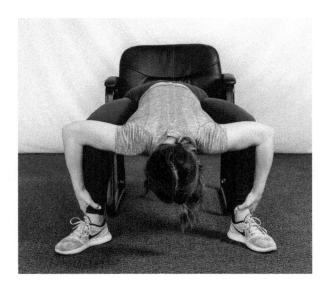

Common mistakes:
- Not sitting on the edge of your chair when performing the stretch
- Not having your legs far enough apart, thus effectively blocking your torso from leaning down

Lumbar Flexion (Supine)

Starting position: Lie on your back and comfortably bend both knees.

The movement: Reach out with your arms and grab your knees (either from over the top of your knees or from underneath your knees). Keep your knees together and pull both knees toward your chest. Hold the end stretch position a couple of seconds, and then return to the starting position.

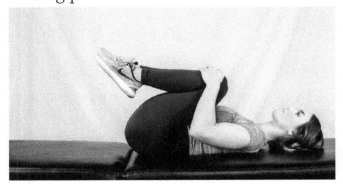 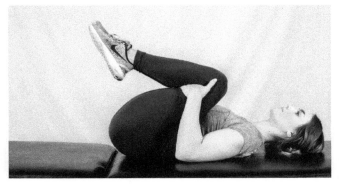

Supported: If reaching for both knees simultaneously is too difficult or painful, then try supported. Wrap a towel under both legs, and grab each end. Use the towel to pull your knees toward your chest.

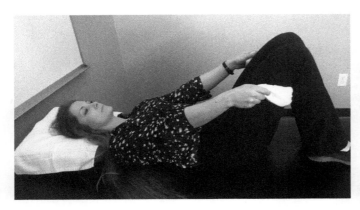 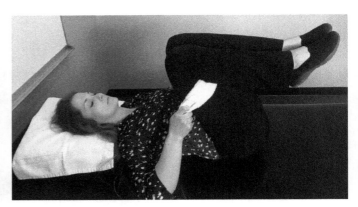

Common mistakes:

*   Leaning torso upward toward your knees
*   Pulling legs outward instead of straight toward the chest

Prone Press-Ups/Cobra Stretch

Starting position: Lie on your stomach (facedown). Place your hands by your side/shoulders in a comfortable position.

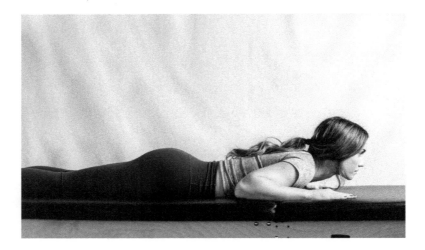

The movement: Keep your hips relaxed and push upward by straightening your elbows. Hold the stretch at the end position for a couple of seconds, and then return to the starting position.

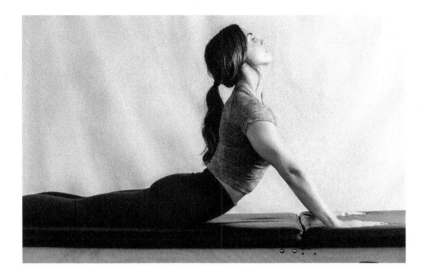

Common mistakes:

- Lifting your hips off the floor/bed as you stretch upward (i.e., planking)
- Placing your hands too low (closer to the hips) so that the elbows are not allowed to fully straighten during the stretch
- Tightening your hips/buttocks during the stretch (should remain relaxed throughout)

Elbow Press-Ups

If the prone press-up stretch is too challenging or painful, elbow press-ups are a good alternative stretch to perform.

Starting position: Modify the starting position on your stomach so that your arms are under the shoulders and forearms are on the floor.

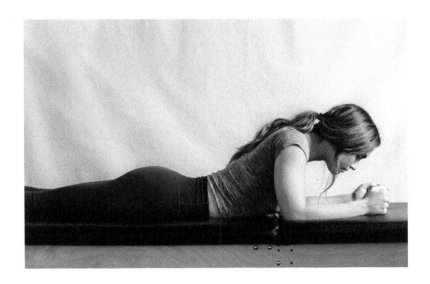

The movement: Keep your hips relaxed and push upward using your forearms. Hold the end stretch position a couple of seconds, and then return to the starting position (your elbows may or may not fully straighten depending on the stiffness of the stretch).

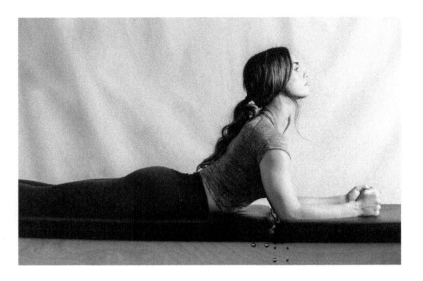

Common mistakes:
- Lifting your hips upward (planking) during the movement
- Tightening up your buttocks/hips during the movement (should remain relaxed throughout the movement)

Hamstring Stretch

Starting position: Lie on your back with your legs straight and loop a towel/belt/strap around the forefoot area.

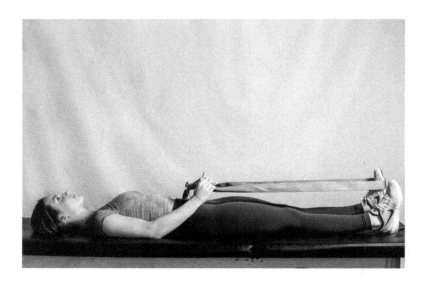

The movement: Use the strap to pull your foot/leg upward toward the ceiling while keeping your knee fully straight. Hold the end stretch position for a couple of seconds, and then return to the starting position. The opposite leg should remain fully straight during the stretch.

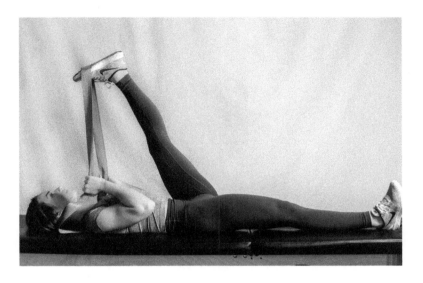

Common mistakes:
- Bending the knee as you perform the hamstring stretch.
- Using a stretch band instead of a strap/belt/towel. The band will stretch, and the hamstrings will not.
- Bending the opposite leg during the stretch

Ankle/Calf Stretch

Starting position: In standing, lean your forearms up against a wall, and shift one leg forward and one leg backward. The backward leg will be the leg getting the stretch.

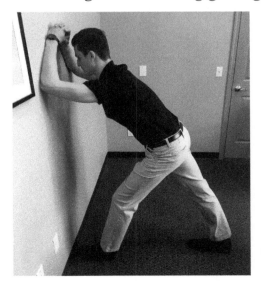

The movement: Keep your back heel firmly planted on the floor (and your back knee straight) as you push your forward knee toward the wall. Hold the end stretch position for a couple of seconds, and then return to the starting position.

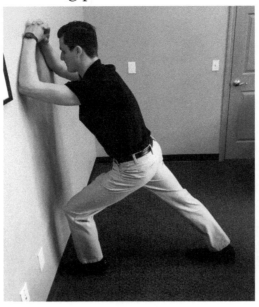

Common mistakes:
- Allowing the back heel to rise off the floor during the stretch.
- Placing the back leg too far back or not far enough back to optimize the stretch.
- Bending the knee of the back leg during the stretch

Shoulder Extension (Doorjamb)

Starting position: Face away from the doorjamb. Reach back and place your hand (thumb down) onto the doorjamb.

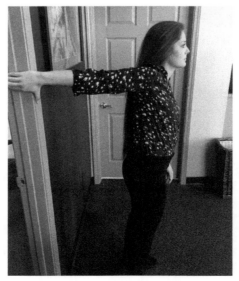

The movement: Keep your hand against the doorjamb, and do a partial/minisquat by bending your knees. Hold the end stretch position for a couple of seconds, and then return to starting position.

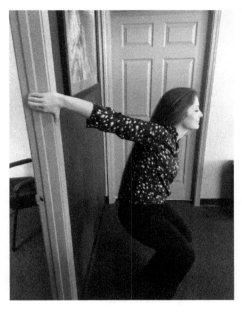

Common mistakes:
- Placing your hand on the wrong side of the doorjamb
- Not placing thumbs pointing downward toward the floor
- Placing hand too high on the doorjamb (unable to squat downward for the stretch)
- Placing hand too low on the doorjamb (have to squat way down to feel the stretch)

Chapter 15

Eleven Ways to Create a Healthy Lifestyle

Now that you have learned what you need to do to "survive" in today's sitting society, it's time to focus on truly improving your physical and mental health. This chapter exists as a reminder that all it takes is a few simple changes to improve your livelihood. Listed below are eleven tips I believe can improve your overall well-being. The next few pages will go into detail about each recommendation and explain how incorporating the change can boost your health both mentally and physically. In other words, how to truly "thrive" in today's sitting society.

1. Take a daily walk.

2. Take up yoga.

3. Take up a lifetime sport, exercise, or movement. Common examples include:
   a. Golf, tennis, pickleball, swimming, biking, hiking, CrossFit, weight training, yoga, skiing, bowling, paddle boarding, kayaking, walking, running, dancing, Tai Chi

4. Drink more water.

5. Practice diaphragmatic breathing, meditation, or tai chi.

6. Get more sleep.

7. Focus on nutritional considerations.

8. Perform daily balance training.

9. Take a daily nap.

10. Stretch daily.

11. Take up weights or resistance training.

1. Take a daily walk.

Walking is an easy exercise that almost every person can do every day. Walking is low impact, requires minimal equipment, can be done at any time of day, and can be performed at your own pace. You can get out and walk without worrying about the risks associated with more vigorous forms of exercise. Walking is also a great form of physical activity for people who are overweight, elderly, or who haven't exercised in a long time. How much walking is needed? Surprisingly, it's not as much as you would think. In a cohort study, 16,741 women with a mean average of 72 years had their steps per day counted over seven days. Women who averaged approximately 4,400 steps per day had significantly lower mortality rates compared with less active women that averaged 2,700 steps per day[104]. The American Heart Association (AHA) recommends at least 150 minutes of moderate physical activity per week. Taking a brisk 30 minute walk five days a week will definitely meet the criteria of moderate physical activity. Many people get dogs as a way to help motivate them to take daily walks. Unfortunately that is not the case with my parents. Sheila (their rescue Australian Shepherd) gets lots of food and no walks ever. Some of the many health benefits of walking include the following:

- Increased cardiovascular and pulmonary (heart and lung) fitness

- Reduced risk of heart disease and stroke

- Improved management of conditions such as hypertension (high blood pressure), high cholesterol, joint and muscular pain or stiffness, and diabetes

- Stronger bones and improved balance

- Increased muscle strength and endurance

- Reduced body fat

- Staying healthier, feeling stronger, living longer

2. Take up yoga.

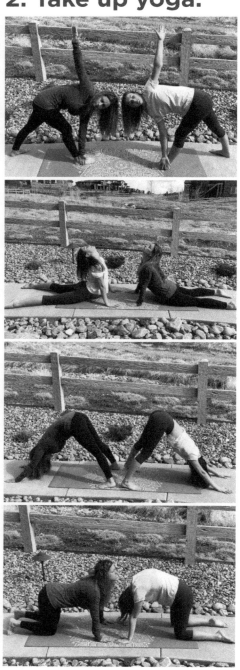

Yoga is another great activity/exercise that can easily be implemented into your everyday life. According to the American Osteopathic Association, regular yoga can provide many physical and mental health benefits. Physical benefits of yoga include the following:

- Increased flexibility

- Increased muscle strength and tone

- Improved respiration, energy, and vitality

- Balanced metabolism

- Lowered blood pressure

- Reduced insomnia

- Reduced headaches

- Decreased chronic spine pain and arthritis pain

- Weight reduction

- Cardiovascular and circulatory health

- Improved athletic performance

- Protection from injury

Many muscles become inhibited by not being used for long periods of time. This may cause you to feel tight and sore at the end of the day. One method to alleviating these symptoms of pain is to try yoga, a practice that has been around for over 2,000 years. Yoga encompasses three components which are body position and posture, breathing, and meditation with a focus on the state of mind.[44] Yoga ranges in difficulty, with easier poses and stretches, to more advanced practices. One common area of pain caused by prolonged sitting is the lower back. Yoga can work on this tension by gently and calmly stretching and strengthening the lower back muscles while increasing blood circulation throughout the body, which can in turn contribute to getting nutrients to injured muscles. The American Osteopathic Association explains that yoga's benefits include not only increased flexibility and strength, but also improved respiration and energy, a stable metabolism, weight loss, protection from future injury, and better cardiovascular and circulatory health.[45]

Mental Benefits of Yoga

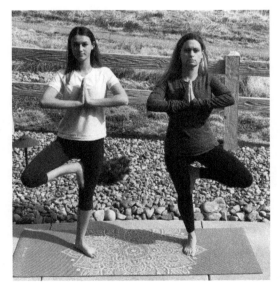

There is a growing body of research to back up yoga's mental health benefits. Yoga increases body awareness, relieves stress, reduces muscle tension, strain, and inflammation, sharpens attention and concentration, and calms and centers the nervous system. Yoga's positive benefits on mental health have made it an important practice tool of psychotherapy.[105] It has been shown to enhance social well-being through a sense of belonging to others, and improve the symptoms of depression, attention deficit and hyperactivity, and sleep disorders. Dr. Natalie Nevins, a doctor of osteopathic medicine and trained yoga instructor, explains the mental benefits of yoga: "Regular yoga practice creates mental clarity and calmness; increases body awareness; relieves chronic stress patterns, relaxes the mind; centers attention; and sharpens concentration."[45] With a focus on breathing throughout the poses, participants will learn where to place their oxygen when inhaling and discover techniques to calm the body during anxiety. Understanding the body is one of the first steps to addressing mental health issues which may rise during long periods of sitting.

Not only can you use yoga to help calm the symptoms that arise from sitting all day, but certain stretches and movements from yoga also can be done throughout the day to alleviate and prevent those symptoms from reoccurring. Examples of these would be head rotations, chin tucks, shoulder rolls, pelvic circles, and back extension.

Upward Facing Dog Benefits
- Reduces stiffness in back
- Improves posture by drawing the shoulders down and back
- Opens up the chest for optimal breathing

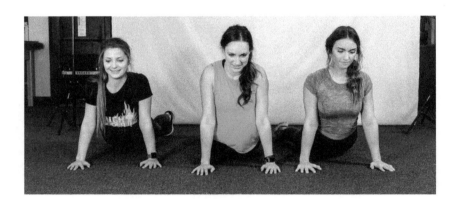

Downward Dog Benefits
- Strengthens the arms, legs, and abs
- Stretches the hamstrings, calves, and muscles of the shoulders

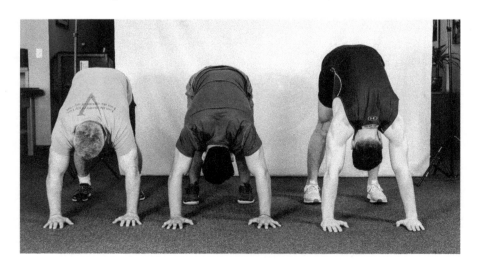

3. Take up a lifetime sport, exercise, or movement.

What is a lifetime sport or lifetime physical activity? It's a sport or physical activity that you can play or do, well, for your entire life. Finding a sport or physical activity you enjoy can greatly improve exercise adherence (maintaining consistent and regular physical activity). It's much easier to find the time, motivation, and even money for sports/physical activity when it is fun and rewarding. Examples of lifetime sports/physical activities include: golf, tennis, pickleball, swimming, walking, biking, hiking, CrossFit, weight training, yoga, skiing, bowling, paddleboarding, kayaking, and running. Exercise physiologist Bob Hopper distilled that advice into a book called *Stick with Exercise for a Lifetime: How to Enjoy Every Minute of It!* His take: "While visions of improved health and fitness—not to mention looking and feeling great—can get most of us started on an exercise program, they're notoriously weak motivators over the long haul," he writes. Instead, he argues, if you "pursue a physical activity program with the goal of having fun, learning new skills, and improving performance," better health and fitness will come along as "natural byproducts."

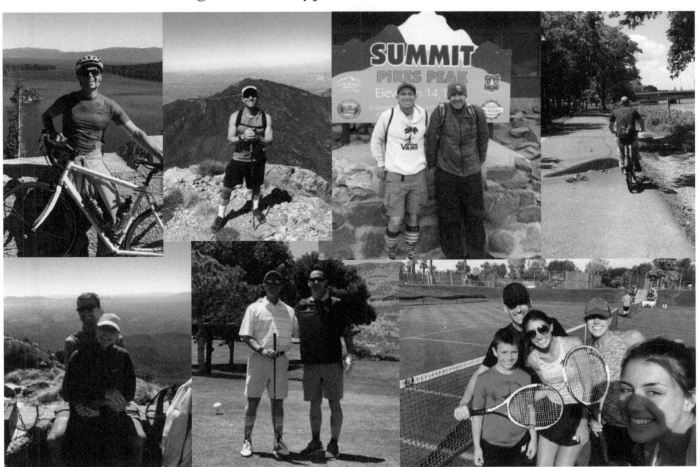

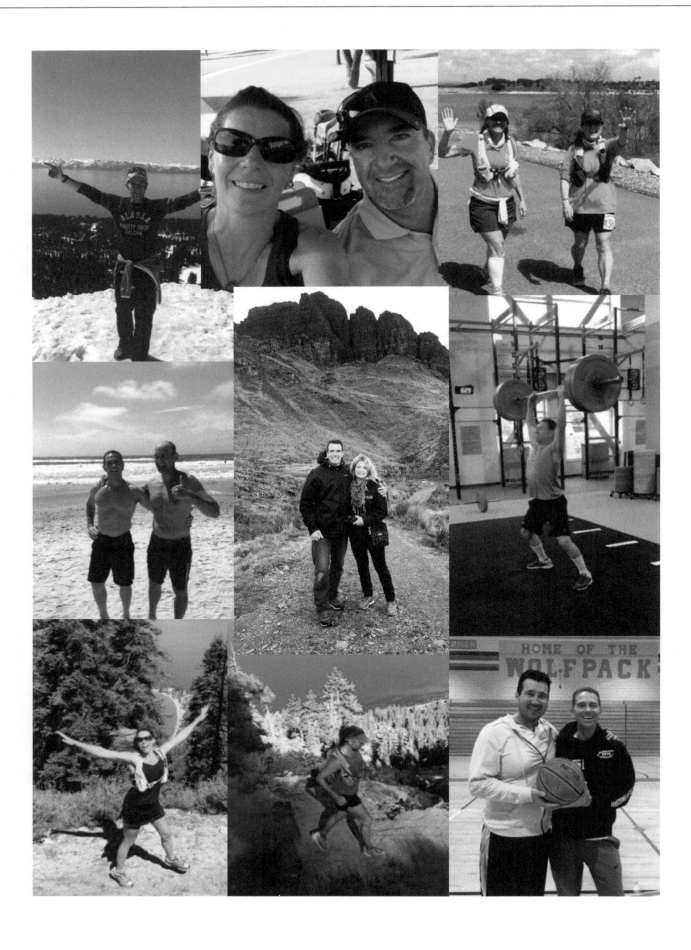

4. Drink more water.

Water is vital to the health and function of every single cell in the body. Even a slight loss of water to a cell can cause significant impairment to the function of a cell as well as cell damage. The general recommendation for adequate water consumption is two liters (64 ounces) per day.

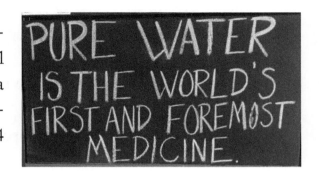

Seven Evidence-Based Health Benefits of Drinking Water

1. **Water helps to maximize physical performance.**

   Your body is made up of 60–70% water. Losing as little as 2% of your body's water content can significantly impair physical performance.

2. **Hydration has a major effect on energy levels and brain function.**

   Your brain is strongly influenced by your hydration status. Studies show that even mild dehydration (1–3% of body weight) can impair many aspects of brain function.

3. **Drinking water may help prevent and treat headaches.**

   Dehydration can trigger headaches and migraines in some individuals. Several studies have shown that water can relieve headaches in those who are dehydrated.

4. **Drinking more water may help relieve constipation.**

   Constipation is a common problem, characterized by infrequent bowel movements and difficulty passing stools. Increasing fluid intake is often recommended as a part of the treatment protocol, and there is some evidence to back this up. Low water consumption appears to be a risk factor for constipation in both young and elderly individuals. Drinking plenty of water can help prevent and relieve constipation, especially in people who generally do not drink enough water.

5. Drinking more water may help treat kidney stones.

Urinary stones are painful clumps of mineral crystal that form in the urinary system. The most common form is kidney stones, which form in the kidneys. There is limited evidence that water intake can help prevent recurrence in people who previously had kidney stones.

6. Water helps prevent hangovers.

A hangover refers to the unpleasant symptoms experienced after drinking alcohol. Alcohol is a diuretic, so it makes you lose more water than you take in. This can lead to dehydration. Although dehydration is not the main cause of hangovers, it can cause symptoms like thirst, fatigue, headache and dry mouth. A good way to reduce hangovers is to drink a glass of water between drinks, and to have at least one big glass of water before going to bed.

7. Drinking more water can help with weight loss.

Drinking plenty of water can help you lose weight. This is due to the fact that water can increase satiety and boost your metabolic rate. In two studies, drinking half a liter (17 ounces) of water was shown to increase metabolism by 24 to 30% for up to 1.5 hours. This means that drinking two liters of water every day can increase your total energy expenditure by nearly 100 calories per day. The timing of water intake is important as well. Drinking water around a half hour before meals seem to be the most effective in making you feel more satiated, so that you eat fewer calories. In one study, dieters who drank half a liter of water before meals lost 44% more weight over a period of twelve weeks. It is actually best to drink water cold, because then the body will use additional energy (calories) to heat the water to body temperature.

5. Practice diaphragmatic breathing.

When the stomach, rather than the chest, expands with inhalation of air, it is called diaphragmic breathing. When this happens, the diaphragm, which is a large sliver of muscle located at the base of the lungs, is contracting. According to the Cleveland Clinic, this form of breathing is to "strengthen the diaphragm, decrease the work of breathing by slowing the breathing rate, decrease oxygen demand, and use less energy and effort to breathe."[99]

Diaphragmic Breathing to Reduce Stress

An article published through the *Journal of Evidence-Based Complementary and Alternative Medicine* explains that engaging in diaphragmic breathing is "relaxing and therapeutic," thus reducing stress levels and overall adverse health issues. To prove this theory, sixteen athletes were observed after an exercise session. Half of these athletes participated in one hour of diaphragmic breathing while concentrating on their breath in a quiet place, and the other half simply spent the hour sitting in a quiet place. The experiment proved that "relaxation induced by diaphragmic breathing increases the antioxidant defense status in athletes after exhaustive exercise." In other words, lower levels of oxidative stress were observed.[97] Exercise increases oxidative stress, as the article explains, so performing diaphragmic breathing after exercise lowers the oxidative stress, thus lowering the overall risk of diseases such as heart disease, hypertension, and rheumatoid arthritis.

How to Perform Diaphragmic Breathing

Source: Cleveland Clinic

> **Step 1:** Lie on a flat surface, such as the floor or a bed, and place one hand on your chest and one hand on your belly just below the ribcage. (Refer to chapter 10 for tips on good lying posture).

> **Step 2:** Breathe in slowly through your nose, feeling your stomach move out against your hand. The hand on the chest should remain as still as possible.

> **Step 3:** Tighten the stomach muscles inward as you exhale. The hand on the chest should continue to remain still.

Continue to practice for five to ten minutes at a time, as comfortable.

6. Get more sleep.

Getting enough sleep improves your health, strengthens your immune system, improves your mood, boosts productivity, and improves brain function; chronic poor sleep is linked to poor health, mood disorders, and low productivity. Improving sleep in various demographics could make a positive impact on one's health.[106] The question is: How much sleep is enough? While sleep requirements vary slightly from person to person, most healthy adults need between seven to nine hours of sleep per night to function at their best. Children and teens need even more. And despite the notion that our sleep needs decrease with age, most older people still need at least seven hours of sleep.[106] More than one-third of American adults are not getting enough sleep on a regular basis, according to a new study in the Centers for Disease Control and Prevention's (CDC) *Morbidity and Mortality Weekly Report*. This is the first study to document estimates of self-reported healthy sleep duration (seven or more hours per day) for all fifty states and the District of Columbia.

Although an individual's sleep needs may vary, studies do show that Americans are not getting enough sleep. And not only do you need to get enough sleep, your sleep needs to be on a regular schedule. This means going to sleep at around the same time every night and getting up at the same time every morning (yes, even on the weekends!). Obesity, diabetes, and high cholesterol are more prevalent among irregular sleepers. A new study has found that not sticking to a regular bedtime and wakeup schedule, and getting different amounts of sleep each night can put a person at higher risk for obesity, high cholesterol, hypertension, high blood sugar and other metabolic disorders.[107] In fact, for every hour of variability in time to bed and time asleep, a person may have up to a 27% greater chance of experiencing a metabolic abnormality.

Tips for Improving Your Nighttime Sleeping

1. Go to bed and wake up on a regular schedule.

2. Turn off TVs, computers, and cell phones before you go to bed.

3. Don't consume caffeine late in the day.

4. Don't sleep too much during the day. My dad complains about his inability to sleep during the night. However, he takes a nap after breakfast, a nap after lunch, and a nap after dinner. Repeated or long day naps will decrease the quantity and quality of your night sleep.

5. Optimize your bedroom environment. Try to minimize external noise, light, and artificial lights from devices like alarm clocks or cell phones. Make sure your bedroom is a quiet, relaxing, clean, and enjoyable place.

6. Set your ideal bedroom temperature. Having too high or too low of temperature can profoundly affect your sleep.

7. Don't eat late in the evening. Late-night eating may negatively impact both sleep quality and the natural release of HGH and melatonin.

8. Exercise regularly, but not right before bed. Exercise is one of the best science-backed ways to improve your sleep and health. It can enhance all aspects of sleep and has been used to reduce symptoms of insomnia. One study on older adults determined that exercise nearly halved the amount of time it took to fall asleep and provided 41 more minutes of sleep. Personally, I need to do some sort of exercise or physical activity every day. On days I don't move as much, both my quality and quantity of sleep definitely suffer.

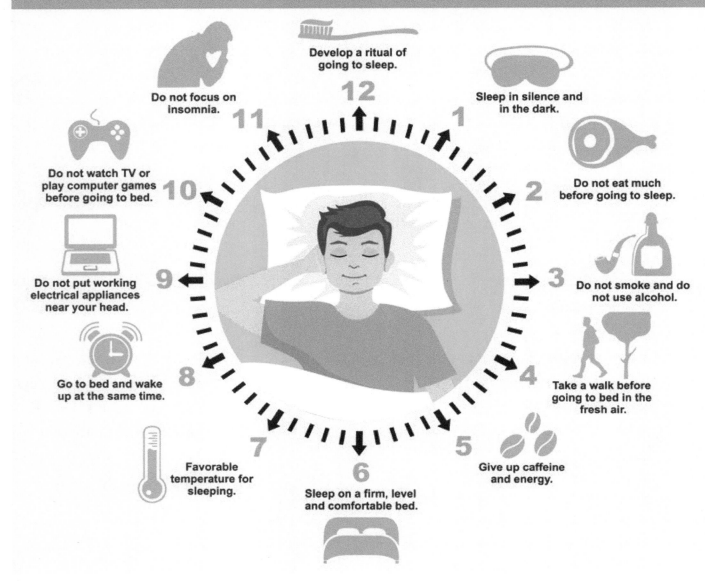

RULES OF HEALTHY SLEEP

Develop a ritual of going to sleep. (12)

Do not focus on insomnia. (11)

Do not watch TV or play computer games before going to bed. (10)

Do not put working electrical appliances near your head. (9)

Go to bed and wake up at the same time. (8)

Favorable temperature for sleeping. (7)

Sleep on a firm, level and comfortable bed. (6)

Give up caffeine and energy. (5)

Take a walk before going to bed in the fresh air. (4)

Do not smoke and do not use alcohol. (3)

Do not eat much before going to sleep. (2)

Sleep in silence and in the dark. (1)

7. Focus on nutritional considerations.

"You are what you eat," the adage says. A whole book can be written about the importance of a healthy diet for your good health and body function. My focus on the topic of nutrition is in the importance of avoiding a diet high in processed foods.

"LET FOOD BE THY MEDICINE AND MEDICINE BE THY FOOD"

Hippocrates

Processed Food and Body Inflammation

Inflammation of the body can be both beneficial and harmful. It can be beneficial through its ability to defend the body from illnesses and its ability to stimulate healing. Chronic and sustained inflammation, on the other hand is linked to disorders such as diabetes, obesity, and heart disease.[108] Interestingly, the foods you eat can have a major impact (either good or bad) on body inflammation.

Here are six foods that contribute to an increase in overall body inflammation:

1. **Sugar and high-fructose corn syrup**

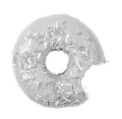

Sugar is 50% glucose and 50% fructose, while high-fructose corn syrup is about 45% glucose and 55% fructose. One of the reasons that added sugars are harmful is that they can increase inflammation, which can lead to disease. Eating a lot of fructose has been linked to obesity, insulin resistance, diabetes, fatty liver disease, cancer, and chronic kidney disease. Food high in added sugar includes candy, chocolate, soft drinks, cakes, cookies, doughnuts, sweet pastries, and certain cereals.

2. **Artificial trans fats**

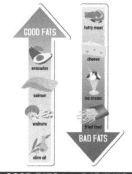

GOOD FATS vs. BAD FATS

Artificial trans fats are likely the unhealthiest fats you can eat. They are created by adding hydrogen to unsaturated fats, which are liquid, in order to give them the stability of a more solid fat. Most margarines contain trans fats, and they are often added to processed foods in order to extend shelf life. Unlike the naturally occurring trans fats found in dairy and meat, artificial trans fats have been shown to cause inflammation and increase disease risk. Foods high in trans fats include french fries and other fried fast food, some varieties of microwave popcorn, certain margarines and vegetable shortening, packaged cakes and cookies, some pastries, and all processed food that lists partially hydrogenated vegetable oil on the label.

3. Vegetable and seed oils

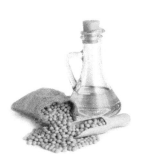

Some scientists believe that certain vegetable oils, such as soybean oil, promote inflammation due to their very high omega-6 fatty acid content. Although some dietary omega-6 fats are necessary, the typical Western diet provides far more than people need. Vegetable and seed oils are used as a cooking oil and are a major ingredient in many processed foods.

4. Refined carbohydrates

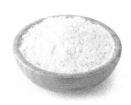

In recent years, carbohydrates have gotten a bad rap (witness all the low carb diet plans that have sprung up in recent years). However, the truth is that not all carbs are bad. There are good carbs, and there are bad carbs. Ancient humans consumed high-fiber, un-processed carbs for millennia in the form of grasses, roots, and fruits. However, eating refined carbs may drive inflammation. Refined carbs have had most of their fiber removed, such as white flour. Fiber promotes fullness, improves blood sugar control, and feeds the beneficial bacteria in your gut. Researchers suggest that the refined carbs in the modern diet may encourage the growth of inflammatory gut bacteria that can increase your risk of obesity and inflammatory bowel disease. Refined carbohydrates are found in candy, bread, pasta, pastries, some cereals, cookies, cakes, sugary soft drinks, and all processed food that contains added sugar or flour.

5. Excessive alcohol

LEAKY GUT

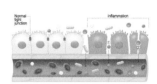

Moderate alcohol consumption has actually been shown to provide some health benefits. However, higher amounts can lead to severe problems. People who drink heavily may develop problems with bacterial toxins moving out of the colon and into the body. This condition—often called "leaky gut"—can drive widespread inflammation that leads to organ damage. Daily recommendations are that adult males should consume no more than two alcoholic beverages per day, while adult females should consume no more than one.

6. Processed meat

Consuming processed meat is associated with an increased risk of heart disease, diabetes, stomach cancer, and colon cancer. Processed meat contains more advanced glycation end products (AGEs) than most other meats. AGEs are formed by cooking meats and some other foods at high temperatures. They are known to cause inflammation. Common types of processed meat include sausage, bacon, ham, smoked meat, and beef jerky.

8. Daily Balance Training

Balance refers to an individual's ability to maintain their line of gravity within their base of support. It can also be described as the ability to maintain equilibrium. Who can benefit from balance training? The answer is everyone! The cost of treating fall-related injuries is among the top 20 for treatment of medical conditions. Falling is the second leading cause of accidental death worldwide and is a major cause of personal injury, especially for the elderly. In fact, the hospital cost of the average fall-related injury is around $30,000. As individuals age, their risk of falling increases dramatically. According to the Centers for Disease Control, individuals who are 65 or older have a 25% chance of falling. The National Council on Aging (NCOA) states that "In 2015, the total cost of fall injuries was $50 billion." Falls account for unintentional injuries, hospital visits, surgery, recovery, and even death. The good news is that many of the falls that people suffer are preventable. Training your balance systems (yes, there are more than one) regularly can definitely decrease your chances of suffering a fall and resultant possible injury. As I often tell my patients "balance is like a muscle," meaning that with regular training, balance will improve and get stronger. There are three main systems involved in achieving good balance, and it is important to train each component to optimize and strengthen your body's ability to stay upright.

1. Visual balance
2. Inner ear (vestibular)
3. Proprioceptive (body awareness)

Visual Balance

Your vision allows you to process information about the environment and thus to help achieve and maintain equilibrium. Problems arise if there is a visual disorder that disrupts the ability of the eye to process this incoming environmental information. However, adults with visual disorders are able to adapt peripheral, vestibular, proprioceptive, and cerebellar processing to help compensate for their visual deficit. As a result, these individuals are often able to achieve and maintain good postural control by training their vestibular and proprioceptive balance systems.

Vestibular Balance

The vestibular system is divided into central (brain and brainstem) and the peripheral system (the inner ear and pathways to the brainstem). Your inner ear is the location of your sensory system that provides a sense of balance and spatial orientation for controlling balance during movement. When disrupted, people often experience dizziness, vertigo (sense of spinning or boat rocking), and other types of disequilibrium. To optimize vestibular balance training, you must first dampen the other balance systems (vison and proprioception), and then focus on training the vestibular system.

Proprioceptive Balance

Proprioception is the medical term that describes the ability to sense the orientation of your body in your environment. It allows you to move quickly and freely without having to consciously think about where you are in space or in your environment. Proprioception comes from sensory nerve endings that provide our brain with the information of the limb position. Examples of proprioception include the awareness of having your arm overhead (even with eyes closed), or the awareness of walking on a sidewalk versus walking in grass.

Daily Balance Training

When you perform balance training, it is important to implement strategies that will effectively train each of the three different balance systems. By implementing the simple balance training strategies below, you will effectively train each of the balance systems, thus optimizing your improvement in your overall balance. A good question to ask right now is "Where do I begin in the progression of balance training?" My suggestion is to start at number one, and if it's too easy, then move to two. If two is too easy, then move to number three. Stop at the number where you are having difficulty or challenge maintaining your balance for more than five to ten seconds. If you get to number eight and it is still easy? Well then you already have extraordinary balance.

When you train balance, safety is vitally important. The last thing you want to do is actually fall while doing balance training. To safely train your balance, have protections in place to stop you from falling if you lose your balance. An example would include having a stable object to easily grab (counter/sink/couch etc.) Another example would be to do your balance training in a narrow hallway where you can easily hold onto the wall if needed.

Balance Training Progression

The bolded words highlight the change/progression from each of the eight balance training exercises.

1. Practice static standing with both feet together, eyes open, and on a flat surface.

2. Practice static standing with both feet together, **eyes closed**, and on a flat surface.

3. Practice static standing with both feet together, **eyes closed, and on an uneven surface.**

4. Practice static standing with both feet together, **eyes closed, on an uneven surface, and while turning your head side to side.**

5. Practice static standing on a **single leg**, eyes open, and on a flat surface.

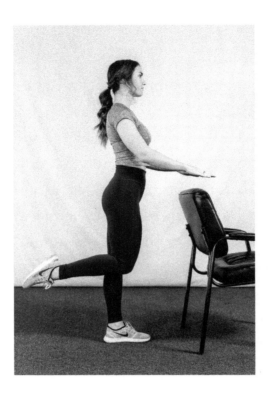

6. Practice static standing on a **single leg**, **eyes closed**, and on a flat surface.

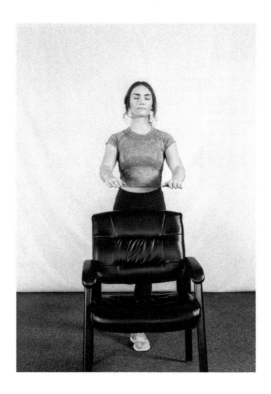

7. Practice static standing on a **single leg, eyes closed, and on an uneven surface.**

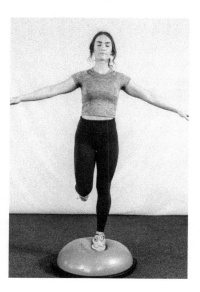

8. Practice static standing on a **single leg, eyes closed, on an uneven surface, and while turning your head side to side.**

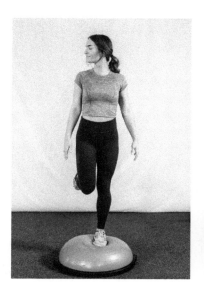 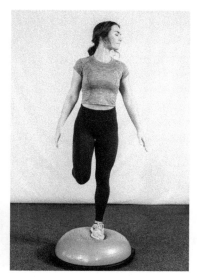

Fall Prevention Programs

The Otago Exercise Program Stay Active and Independent for Lift (SAIL)

Stepping On: Tai Chi for Arthritis

Tai Ji Quan: Moving for Better Balance

YMCA Moving for Better Balance

A Matter of Balance: The Fallscape System

Safe and Steady: Bingocize
CAPABLE: Enhance Fitness
FallsTalk
FallScape
Fit & Strong: Healthy Steps for Older Adults
Healthy Steps in Motion

9. Take a daily nap.

As I often tell my patients, the world would be a better place to live in if everyone took a 20-30 minute nap every day. According to the National Sleep Foundation, the United States appears to be becoming more and more sleep deprived. And it may be our busy lifestyle that keeps us from napping. While naps do not necessarily make up for inadequate or poor quality nighttime sleep, a short nap of 20-30 minutes can help to improve mood, alertness and performance. Nappers are in good company: Winston Churchill, John F. Kennedy, Ronald Reagan, Napoleon, Albert Einstein, Thomas Edison, and George W. Bush are known to have valued an afternoon nap. I personally take a 23 minute nap every day.

Tips for good napping include the following:

- **Keep naps short**. Aim to nap for only between 15-30 minutes.. The longer you nap, the more likely you are to feel groggy afterward. However, young adults might be able to tolerate longer naps. Taking longer naps as well as taking multiple naps a day may also create difficulty with night sleeping.

- **Take naps in the early afternoon.** Napping after 3:00 p.m. can interfere with nighttime sleep. Individual factors, such as your need for sleep, your sleeping schedule, your age, and your medication use can also play a role in determining the best time of day to nap.

- **Create a restful environment**. Nap in a quiet, dark place with a comfortable room temperature and with few distractions.

10. Stretch daily.

"Motion is lotion and rest is rust." This saying is repeated often and much in my clinic. Also, as I learned in physics, Newton's first law states that objects in motion tend to stay in motion, while objects at rest tend to stay at rest. I cannot overstate how important daily stretching/range of motion exercises are for the health of our musculoskeletal system. Stretching daily has many benefits including:

1. Increases your flexibility/range of motion

2. Improves your performance in physical activities

3. Increases blood flow to your muscles

4. Improves your posture

5. Is great for stress relief

6. Can calm your mind

7. Helps decrease tension headaches

Can stretching prevent injury? Several authors have suggested that stretching has a beneficial effect on injury prevention. In contrast, clinical evidence suggesting that stretching before exercise does not prevent injuries has also been reported. Apparently, no scientifically based prescription for stretching exercises exists and no conclusive statements can be made about the relationship of stretching and athletic injuries.[109] That said, in my 17 years practicing as a physical therapist, stretching can magically make pain and injury disappear, as well as help prevent future pain and injury. I can definitively say that stiffness is the enemy of the human musculoskeletal system.

The stretching exercises in this section represent (based on the effects of chronic sitting on joint stiffness as well as my experience as a physical therapist) the single best stretch for each of the major joints negatively affected by sitting. In other words, these daily stretching exercises give you the most "bang for your buck" to help in your fight against joint pain and stiffness caused by chronic sitting. A detailed explanation of each of these stretches can be found in chapters 11 and 14.

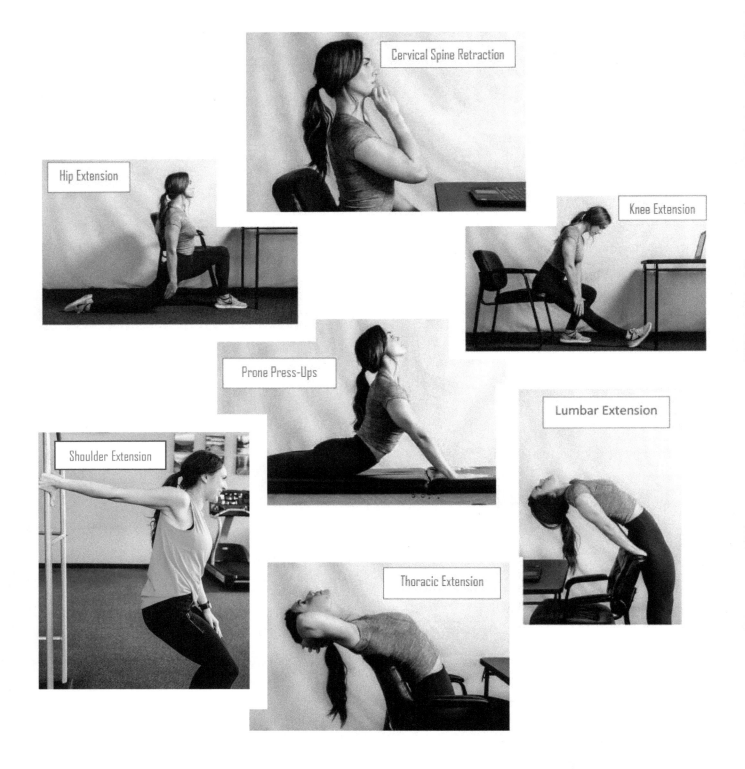

11. Take up weights or resistance training.

Physical Benefits

As I also tell my patients, "Resistance training is medicine for the body and the soul." The benefits of regular resistance training are numerous and many. Study after study purports the many physical and mental benefits associated with a regular resistance training program. Benefits of resistance training include improved physical performance, movement control, walking speed, functional independence, cognitive abilities, and self-esteem. Resistance training may assist in prevention and management of type 2 diabetes by decreasing visceral fat, increasing the density of glucose transporter type 4, and improving insulin sensitivity. Resistance training may enhance cardiovascular health, by reducing resting blood pressure, decreasing low-density lipoprotein cholesterol and triglycerides, and increasing high-density lipoprotein cholesterol. Resistance training may promote bone development, with studies showing a 1 to 3% increase in bone mineral density. Resistance training may also be effective for reducing low back pain and easing discomfort associated with arthritis and fibromyalgia, and has been shown to reverse specific aging factors in Skeletal muscle. Finally, as my CrossFit friends tell me "it makes it a lot harder for you to be killed."

Mental Benefits

The *New York Times* published an article on the benefits of weightlifting for preventing and decreasing depression. The article presented data gathered from over 30 different studies that researchers analyzed. Their findings showed clearly that consistent resistance training, whether heavy or light, anywhere from two to five days per week, helped men and women, young and old alike, to stave off depression and decrease its symptoms. Additionally, weight training was reported to make participants feel immediately better after completing a workout. The article noted that research on the psychological benefits of cardiovascular training, like running and cycling, have long been recommended by the medical community to curb symptoms of many mental illnesses, but an analysis like this—of how weight training affects a mental health condition—is big news.

I began weight-training the day I turned 19 years old, and I continue it today. For me, weight-training changed my body, my mind, and my soul. Prior to starting weight-training, I suffered from poor body image and poor self-esteem. I was very self-conscious about how skinny I was, and felt very unattractive (both inside and outside). Once my body began to change, my mind changed as well. My self-esteem and self-confidence grew exponentially. Without weight-training, I doubt that I would be the same confident, happy, and healthy person that I am today. I simply cannot imagine going through life without both the physical and mental benefits of weight-training.

Some important strengthening exercises that can be incorporated into an exercise regimen are listed below. The next few pages go into detail about how to perform each exercise correctly, as well as how do proper exercise progression.

1. Squats
2. Lunges
3. Dead Lift

4. Bridges
5. Chair dips
6. Push-ups

7. Heel/toe raises
8. Box steps
9. Shoulder press

1. Squats

Target muscles: Gluteus maximus, quadriceps, hamstrings

Starting position: Stand with your feet about hip width apart. Your weight should be more on your heels, and your feet should be slightly turned outward. Tighten your core and keep the inward curve of your low back.

The movement: Keep your weight centered over your heels, and squat down by bending your knees and pushing your hips back. Your knees should stay centered over your feet during the entire movement. Hold the end squat position a couple of seconds, and then return to the starting position.

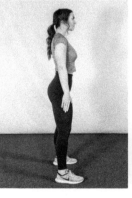 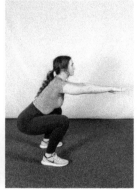

Movement progression: You can progress this exercise by carrying dumbbells in your hands (progressively increasing weight) as you do the squat.

Common mistakes:
- Rounding lower back as you do the movement
- Putting your weight on the balls of your feet during the movement

- Moving knees forward instead of pushing your hips back during the movement
- Not turning feet slightly outward
- Not keeping knees over your feet and letting them move inward during the movement

Squat with Chair

If you are unable to do a full squat (or find it too challenging), try placing a chair behind you. The chair will make the squat movement a little easier, while also training you to push your hips back and keep the weight in the heels. Once you feel the chair, stand back up.

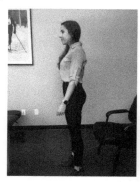
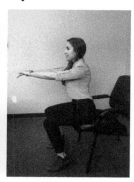

2. Lunges

Target muscles: Gluteus maximus, hamstrings, quadriceps

Starting position: Stand with your feet comfortably apart.

The movement: Take a full step forward, and then lower your hips toward the ground by bending both your forward and back knees. Hold the bottom position a couple of seconds, and then return to the starting position by straightening both your knees and then stepping back. Repeat on the other leg.

Unsupported   *Supported*

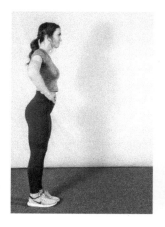
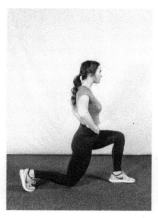
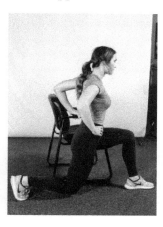

Movement progression: You can progress this exercise by carrying dumbbells in your hands (progressively increasing weight) as you do the lunge.

Common mistakes:
- Not taking a long enough forward step
- Moving knees forward as you lower your hips
- Bending torso forward during the movement (focus on keeping torso fully upright)

3. Dead Lift

Target muscles: Gluteus maximus, hamstrings, quadriceps, erector spinae muscles

Starting position: Bend down by pushing your hips back and bending your knees. Reach for the weight and place your hands securely under the weight/object. Keep your core tight and your low back in lordosis (inward curve).

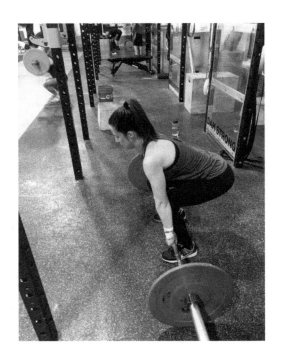

The movement: Lift the weight/object by pushing through your heels, straightening your knees and moving your torso to a fully upright position. Hold for a couple of seconds, and then return to the starting position. All throughout the movement, keep your core tight and low back in lordosis (inward curve).

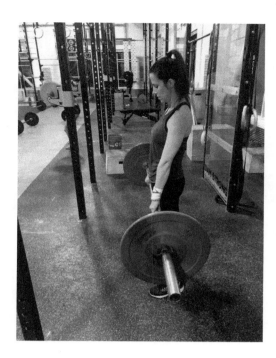

Movement progression: You can progress this exercise by progressively increasing the weight being lifted.

Common mistakes:
- Rounding of lower back (losing inward curve) during the movement
- Bending knees forward instead of pushing hips back during the movement
- Not keeping the object/weight close to your body during the movement
- Putting more of your weight on your forefeet rather than your heels during the lift

4. Bridges

Target muscles: Gluteus maximus, hamstrings, erector spinae muscles, abdominals

Starting position: Lie on your back with your knees comfortably bent and about hip width apart.

The movement: Tighten your abs/core by drawing your naval/belly button inward for bracing. Keep your feet flat, and lift your hips off the floor/mat/bed so that your hips align with your torso. Hold this position for a couple of seconds and then return to the starting position.

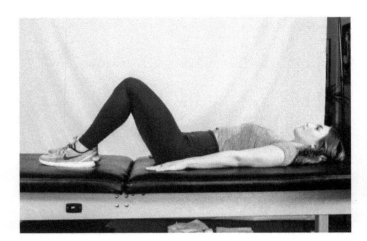
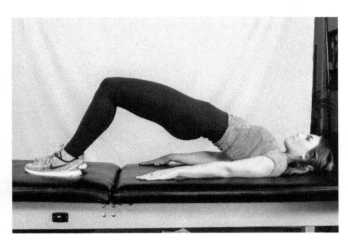

Movement progression: To increase the difficulty of the bridge, you may perform a single leg bridge by keeping one leg fully straight and using the other leg to perform the movement. Alternately, you may hold dumbbells on your hips/thighs as you perform the movement.

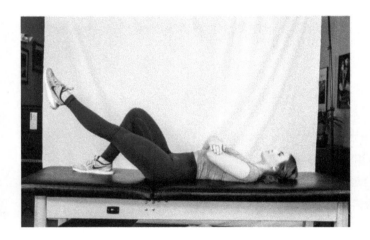
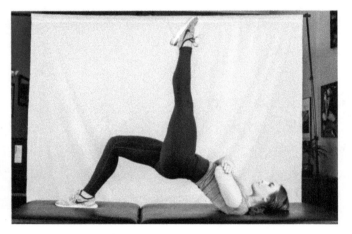

Common mistakes:
- Not tightening your abdominals during the movement
- Either lifting the hips too high or too low (only raise hips to the point of alignment with the torso)
- Not keeping your feet flat during the movement (rising onto the toes)

5. Chair Dips

Target muscles: Triceps, pectoral muscles, deltoid

Starting position: Sit comfortably in a chair with your hands holding onto the armrests.

The movement: Lift your hips off the chair by pushing your hands into the armrests and straightening your elbows. Hold the top position for a couple of seconds, and then return to the starting position. As needed, you may use your legs to assist with performing the movement.

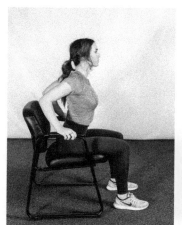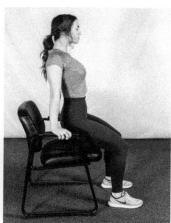

Movement progression: You can increase the difficulty of the movement by using less and less of your legs for assistance, until potentially not using your legs at all.

Common mistakes:
- Using your legs too much during the exercise
- Not using your legs enough (unable to lift hips off the chair)
- Not fully straightening your elbows

6. Angled Push-Ups/Push-Ups
Angled Push-Ups

Target muscles: Pectoral muscles, triceps, deltoids

Starting position: Lean forward over a counter/sink/chair/couch, and place your hands about shoulder width apart and your your elbows straight.

The movement: Keeping your body straight and your core tight, slowly lower your body by bending both your elbows. Then slowly return to the starting position by fully straightening your elbows.

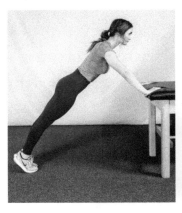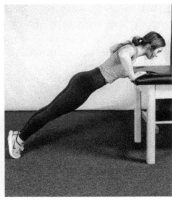

Common mistakes:
- Selecting too low a counter/sink/etc. to lean against (unable to perform the push-up movements)
- Selecting too high a counter/sink/etc. to lean against (too easy to do the push-up movement)
- Not keeping your body straight during the movement
- Not fully bending or straightening your elbows during the movement

Angled Push-Ups Progression: Floor Push-Ups

Movement: As the angled push-ups get easier and easier, you can increase the difficulty of the movement by selecting lower and lower objects to "angle" against, including all the way down to the floor. Floor progression includes knees on floor (easier), and feet on the floor (more difficult).

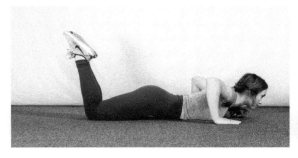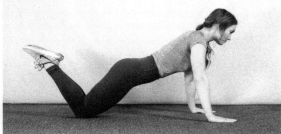

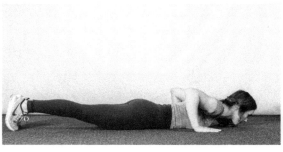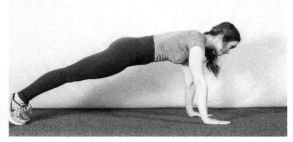

7. Heel/Toe Raises

Target muscles: Gastroc/soleus complex (calves) and shin/pre-tibial muscles

Starting position: Stand comfortably upright with your feet flat on the floor and about hip width apart. Hold onto counter/chair/couch for balance and stability.

The movement: Keep even weight on your legs, and then alternately lift both heels up and then lift up your toes/forefeet.

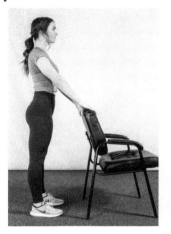 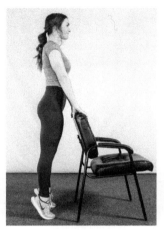 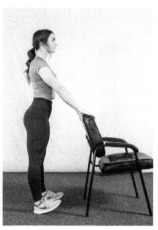

Common mistakes:
- Not holding onto object for stability/balance during the movement
- Not lifting heels or forefeet fully upward
- Not keeping weight evenly distributed during the movement

Movement progression: Lift one leg off the ground, and perform the movement with one leg at a time. You may hold a weight at your side in one hand as you perform the movement with only one leg for further progression.

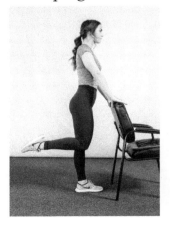 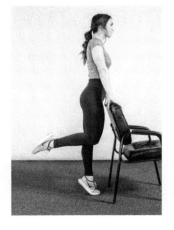 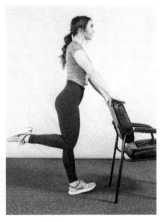

8. Box Steps

Target muscles: Quadriceps, glutes, hamstrings, calves

Starting position: Stand comfortably upright facing your box with feet about hip width apart.

The movement: Step fully onto the box with one foot, and then step fully onto the box with the other foot. Then return to the starting position by stepping down first with one foot and then the other foot. Repeat by alternately stepping up with each foot.

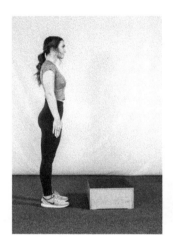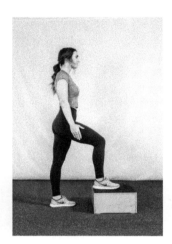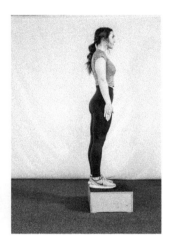

Movement progression: To increase difficulty, step up and down at a faster speed. Another way to progress would be to increase the height of the step so that you would be stepping up higher. A third way to progress would be to hold weights in each of your hands at your side while stepping up and down. Each of these progressions can be done individually or combined.

Common mistakes:
- Not stepping fully upright onto the box
- Not alternating back and forth between left leg and right leg

9. Shoulder Press

Target muscles: Deltoid, pectorals, trapezius, triceps

Starting position: Stand comfortably fully upright with your feet about hip width apart. Bring your weight up to shoulder level by bending your elbows and placing your hands just above your shoulders.

The movement: Press the weight fully over your head by lifting your arms and fully straightening your elbows. Hold for a couple of seconds and then slowly return to the starting position.

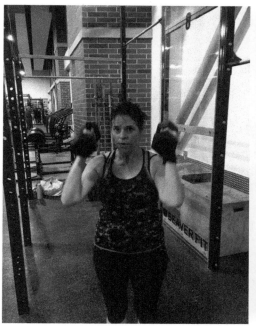 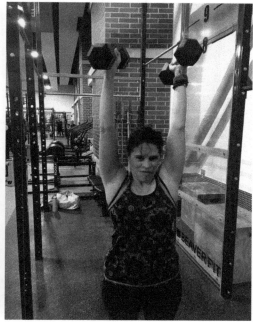

Movement progression: To increase the difficulty of the exercise, try increasing the weights being pressed overhead.

Common mistakes:
- Not fully straightening your elbows as you press the weight over your head
- Pushing the weight forward as you push the weight over your head (focus on pressing the weight straight up over your head)

References

1. Starrett, K. (2016). *Deskbound: Sitting Is the New Smoking*. Victory Belt Publishing. Las Vegas, Nv.

2. Pronk, N. P., Katz, A. S., Lowry, M., & Payfer, J. R. (2012). Reducing occupational sitting time and improving worker health: The Take-a-Stand Project, 2011. *Preventing chronic disease*, *9*, E154.

3. Wheeler, M. J., Dempsey, P. C., Grace, M. S., Ellis, K. A., Gardiner, P. A., Green, D. J., & Dunstan, D. W. (2017). Sedentary behavior as a risk factor for cognitive decline? A focus on the influence of glycemic control in brain health. *Alzheimer's & dementia (New York, N. Y.)*, *3*(3), 291–300. doi:10.1016/j.trci.2017.04.001

4. Perlmuter, L. C., Flanagan, B. P., Shah, P. H., & Singh, S. P. (2009). Glycemic Control and Hypoglycemia: Is the Loser the Winner? Response to Clark. *Diabetes Care*, *31*(10), 2072–2076. doi:10.2337/dc08-2199

5. Ludlow, A. T., Zimmerman, J. B., Witkowski, S., Hearn, J. W., Hatfield, B. D., & Roth, S. M. (2008). Relationship between physical activity level, telomere length, and telomerase activity. *Medicine and science in sports and exercise*, *40*(10), 1764–71.

6. Shammas M. A. (2011). Telomeres, lifestyle, cancer, and aging. *Current opinion in clinical nutrition and metabolic care*, *14*(1), 28–34.

7. The Facts: The Human Body is Designed to Move. Retrieved from https://www.just-stand.org/the-facts/

8.   Waxenbaum J. A., Futterman B. (2019). Anatomy, Back, Intervertebral Discs. [Updated 2018 Dec 13]. In: StatPearls [Internet]. Treasure Island (FL): StatPearls Publishing. Available from: https://www.ncbi.nlm.nih.gov/books/NBK470583/

9.   Ipsos. (2010, August 19). Three out of Four Full-Time Employees of Large Companies Wish They Didn't Spend Most of Their Working Hours Sitting. Retrieved from https://www.ipsos.com/en-us/three-out-four-full-time-employees-large-companies-wish-they-didnt-spend-most-their-working-hours

10.   Held, J. (2015, February 18). How Sitting Ruins the Body (And What You Can Do to Fix It): The Freelancer, by Contently. Retrieved from https://contently.net/2015/02/18/resources/sitting-ruins-body-can-fix/

11.   Bathina, S., & Das, U. N. (2015). Brain-derived neurotrophic factor and its clinical implications. *Archives of medical science: AMS, 11*(6), 1164–78.

12.   Schmolesky, M. T., Webb, D. L., & Hansen, R. A. (2013). The effects of aerobic exercise intensity and duration on levels of brain-derived neurotrophic factor in healthy men. *Journal of sports science & medicine, 12*(3), 502–11.

13.   Katzman, W. B., Wanek, L., Shepherd, J. A., & Sellmeyer, D. E. (2010). Age-related hyperkyphosis: its causes, consequences, and management. *The Journal of orthopaedic and sports physical therapy, 40*(6), 352–60.

14.   Lis, A. M., Black, K. M., Korn, H., & Nordin, M. (2006). Association between sitting and occupational LBP. *European spine journal: official publication of the European Spine Society, the European Spinal Deformity Society, and the European Section of the Cervical Spine Research Society, 16*(2), 283–98.

15.   Teychenne, M., Costigan, S. A., & Parker, K. (2015). The association between sedentary behaviour and risk of anxiety: a systematic review. *BMC public health, 15*, 513. doi:10.1186/s12889-015-1843-x

16. SitFlow. (2018, January 30). 10 Side Effects of Sitting All Day. Retrieved August 16, 2019, from https://hovrpro.com/blogs/news/10-side-effects-of-sitting-all-day

17. Motion Therapy. (2017, July 10). Sitting Disease Statistics. Retrieved August 16, 2019, from https://motiontherapy.net/sitting-disease-statistics/

18. Nielsen. (2014, May 27). Multi-Platform Gaming: For the Win! Retrieved August 16, 2019, from https://www.nielsen.com/us/en/insights/news/2014/multi-platform-gaming-for-the-win.html

19. Roberts, J. D., Rodkey, L., Ray, R., Knight, B., & Saelens, B. E. (2017). Electronic media time and sedentary behaviors in children: Findings from the Built Environment and Active Play Study in the Washington DC area. *Preventive medicine reports*, *6*, 149–156. doi:10.1016/j.pmedr.2017.02.021

20. Du M. (2017). Do Our Cells Pay the Price When We Sit Too Much? *American journal of public health*, *107*(9), 1360–1362.

21. Hall, H. (2014, November 25). Product B: Here We Go Again. Retrieved August 16, 2019, from https://sciencebasedmedicine.org/product-b-here-we-go-again/

22. Boccardi, V., Paolisso, G., & Mecocci, P. (2016). Nutrition and lifestyle in healthy aging: the telomerase challenge. *Aging*, *8*(1), 12–5.

23. Arsenis, N. C., You, T., Ogawa, E. F., Tinsley, G. M., & Zuo, L. (2017). Physical activity and telomere length: Impact of aging and potential mechanisms of action. *Oncotarget*, *8*(27), 45008–45019.

24. Park, Y., & Bae, Y. (2014). Comparison of postures according to sitting time with the leg crossed. *Journal of physical therapy science*, *26*(11), 1749–52.

25. Ding, D., Gebel, K., Phongsavan, P., Bauman, A. E., & Merom, D. (2014). Driving: a road to unhealthy lifestyles and poor health outcomes. *PloS one*, *9*(6), e94602. doi:10.1371/journal.pone.0094602

26. Tenebruso, J. (2017, February 25). 21 Video Game Stats That Will Blow You Away. Retrieved August 16, 2019, from https://www.fool.com/investing/2017/02/25/21-video-game-stats-that-will-blow-you-away.aspx

27. NFPT Team. (2015, February 13). Connective Tissue Training. Retrieved August 16, 2019, from https://www.nfpt.com/blog/connective-tissue-training

28. Bau, J. G., Chia, T., Wei, S. H., Li, Y. H., & Kuo, F. C. (2017). Correlations of Neck/Shoulder Perfusion Characteristics and Pain Symptoms of the Female Office Workers with Sedentary Lifestyle. *PloS one*, *12*(1), e0169318. doi:10.1371/journal.pone.0169318

29. Burke, K. (2016, May 24). 107 Texting Statistics That Answer All Your Questions. Retrieved August 16, 2019, from https://www.textrequest.com/blog/texting-statistics-answer-questions/

30. Shoshany, S., DC, CCEP. (2015, November 6). A Modern Spine Ailment: Text Neck. Retrieved August 7, 2019, from https://www.spine-health.com/blog/modern-spine-ailment-text-neck

31. Neupane, S., Ali, U. T. I., & A, M. (2017). Text Neck Syndrome-Systematic Review. Imperial Journal of Interdisciplinary Research, 3(7), 141–148. Retrieved from https://www.academia.edu/34770472/Text_Neck_Syndrome_-Systematic_Review

32. Davis D, Vasudevan A. Sciatica. [Updated 2019 Feb 28]. In: StatPearls [Internet]. Treasure Island (FL): StatPearls Publishing. Available from: https://www.ncbi.nlm.nih.gov/books/NBK507908/

33. Volpon J. B. (2016). Femoroacetabular impingement. *Revista brasileira de ortopedia*, *51*(6), 621–629. doi:10.1016/j.rboe.2016.10.006

34. Cleveland Clinic. (n.d.). Degenerative Back Conditions. Retrieved August 16, 2019, from https://my.clevelandclinic.org/health/diseases/16912-degenerative-back-conditions

35. Mayo Clinic. (2018, March 06). Herniated disk. Retrieved August 21, 2019, from https://www.mayoclinic.org/diseases-conditions/herniated-disk/symptoms-causes/syc-20354095

36. Lee, N. K., Jung, S. I., Lee, D. Y., & Kang, K. W. (2017). Effects of Exercise on Cervical Angle and Respiratory Function in Smartphone Users. *Osong public health and research perspectives*, *8*(4), 271–274. doi:10.24171/j.phrp.2017.8.4.07

37. Uhlig, S. E., Marchesi, L. M., Duarte, H., & Araújo, M. T. (2015). Association between respiratory and postural adaptations and self-perception of school-aged children with mouth breathing in relation to their quality of life. *Brazilian journal of physical therapy*, *19*(3), 201–10.

38. Fox, A., Bedi, A., Rodeo, S. (2009, November 2). The Basic Science of Articular Cartilage. Structure, Composition, and Function. *Sports Health Journal*. 1(6), 461-468.

39. Salmon, J., & Okely, T. (2011). Sitting Less for Children. Retrieved from https://www.heartfoundation.org.au/images/uploads/publications/PA-Sitting-Less-Child.pdf

40. Benefits of Sitting vs. Standing for Children. (2017, December 22). Retrieved August 7, 2019, from https://www.startstanding.org/sitting-vs-standing-for-children/

41. North Shore Pediatric Therapy. (2017, September 20). W-Sitting And Your Child's Growth. Retrieved August 7, 2019, from https://nspt4kids.com/parenting/w-sitting-and-your-childs-growth/

42.   Shoshany, S. (2015, November 6). A Modern Spine Ailment: Text Neck. Retrieved from https://www.spine-health.com/blog/modern-spine-ailment-text-neck

43.   Young, B. (2018, September 18). Upper Crossed Syndrome. Retrieved August 7, 2019, from https://www.healthline.com/health/upper-crossed-syndrome

44.   Busch, F. (2004, January 27). Healing Benefits of Yoga. Retrieved August 7, 2019, from https://www.spine-health.com/wellness/yoga-pilates-tai-chi/healing-benefits-yoga

45.   American Osteopathic Association. (n.d.). Benefits of Yoga. Retrieved August 7, 2019, from https://osteopathic.org/what-is-osteopathic-medicine/benefits-of-yoga/

46.   Johns Hopkins Medicine. (n.d.). Varicose Veins. Retrieved August 14, 2019, from https://www.hopkinsmedicine.org/healthlibrary/conditions/cardiovascular_diseases/varicose_veins_85,p08259

47.   NHS. (2017, October 31). How Can I Speed up my Metabolism? Retrieved August 21, 2019, from https://www.nhs.uk/live-well/healthy-weight/metabolism-and-weight-loss/

48.   Cleveland Clinic. (2019, April 16). Back Health and Posture. Retrieved August 14, 2019, from https://my.clevelandclinic.org/health/articles/4485-back-health--posture

49.   Triano, J., & Selby, N. C. (2006, September 26). Office Chair, Posture, and Driving Ergonomics. Retrieved August 14, 2019, from https://www.spine-health.com/wellness/ergonomics/office-chair-posture-and-driving-ergonomics

50.   American Chiropractic Association. (n.d.). Maintaining Good Posture. Retrieved August 14, 2019, from https://acatoday.org/content/posture-power-how-to-correct-your-body-alignment

51.   Harvard Health Publishing. (n.d.). 4 ways to turn good posture into less back pain. Retrieved August 7, 2019, from https://www.health.harvard.edu/pain/4-ways-to-turn-good-posture-into-less-back-pain

52.   Shippee, M. (2018, October 26). Stand Up for Good Posture. Retrieved August 7, 2019, from https://www.paleoplan.com/2017/01-04/stand-up-for-good-posture/

53.   Maciałczyk-Paprocka, K., Stawi ska-Witoszy ska, B., Kotwicki, T., Sowi ska, A., Krzy aniak, A., Walkowiak, J., & Krzywi ska-Wiewiorowska, M. (2017). Prevalence of incorrect body posture in children and adolescents with overweight and obesity. *European journal of pediatrics*, *176*(5), 563–572.

54.   Avoiding Shoulder Pain at Work. (2016, December 16). Retrieved from https://www.healthline.com/health/chronic-pain/shoulder-pain-at-work

55.   The National Sleep Foundation. (n.d.). Which Sleep Position is the Best? Retrieved August 7, 2019, from https://www.sleep.org/articles/best-sleep-position/

56.   Argosy Publishing, Inc. (n.d.). Joints and Ligaments: Types of Joints in the Human Body. Retrieved August 7, 2019, from https://www.visiblebody.com/learn/skeleton/joints-and-ligaments

57.   Benney, E. (2017, October 6). How Posture Might Impact a Child's Development. Retrieved August 14, 2019, from https://pyramidprek.com/how-posture-might-impact-a-childs-development/

58.   Cleveland Clinic. (2019, April 13). Metabolic Syndrome. Retrieved August 14, 2019, from https://my.clevelandclinic.org/health/diseases/10783-metabolic-syndrome

59.   National Heart, Lung, and Blood Institute. (n.d.). Metabolic Syndrome. Retrieved August 14, 2019, from https://www.nhlbi.nih.gov/health-topics/metabolic-syndrome

60. Garikiparithi, M. (2017, July 18). Dowager's Hump (Kyphosis): Causes, Symptoms, Treatment & Exercises. Retrieved August 14, 2019, from https://www.belmarrahealth.com/dowager-hump-kyphosis/

61. American Posture Institute. (2016, February 11). Forward Head Posture, a Corporate Nightmare. Retrieved August 14, 2019, from https://americanpostureinstitute.com/forward-head-posture-a-corporate-nightmare/

62. Shaghayegh fard, B., Ahmadi, A., Maroufi, N. et al. (2016). Evaluation of Forward Head Posture in Sitting and Standing Positions. *European Spine Journal*, *25* (11), 3577–3582. https://doi.org/10.1007/s00586-015-4254-x

63. MUSC Health. (n.d.). Posture Change With Age. Retrieved August 14, 2019, from https://muschealth.org/medical-services/geriatrics-and-aging/healthy-aging/posture

64. Drzał-Grabiec, J., Snela, S., Rykała, J., Podgórska, J., & Bana , A. (2013). Changes in the body posture of women occurring with age. *BMC geriatrics*, *13*, 108. doi:10.1186/1471-2318-13-108

65. Wong, M. (2019, May 31). How to fix your Hyperlordosis (Arched back). Retrieved August 21, 2019, from http://posturedirect.com/fix-hyperlordosis-arched-back/

66. Zhang, Y. G., Guo, T. M., Guo, X., & Wu, S. X. (2009). Clinical diagnosis for discogenic low back pain. *International journal of biological sciences*, *5*(7), 647–58.

67. National Spine and Pain Centers. (n.d.). Discogenic Back Pain. Retrieved August 21, 2019, from https://treatingpain.com/condition/discogenic-back-pain

68. Levy, J. (2017, June 13). Pronation Problems: Signs, Causes, and Ways to Correct These Common Posture Problems. Retrieved August 21, 2019, from https://draxe.com/pronation/#

69. Kang, S. (2017). The use of body mechanics principle, clinical-practice fatigue, and practice satisfaction of nursing students. *NursingPlus Open, 3*, 6–10. doi:10.1016/j.npls.2017.03.001

70. Bailey, A. (2017, November 21). Four Basic Principles of Body Mechanics. Retrieved August 21, 2019, from https://healthyliving.azcentral.com/four-basic-principles-body-mechanics-1730.html

71. ACE Physical Therapy and Sports Medicine Institute. (2018, March 13). Push or Pull When Moving Heavy Objects? Retrieved August 21, 2019, from http://www.ace-pt.org/push-or-pull-when-moving-heavy-objects/

72. URMC. (n.d.). The Right Way to Push and Pull. Retrieved August 21, 2019, from https://www.urmc.rochester.edu/encyclopedia/content.aspx?contenttypeid=1&contentid=4458

73. UAH. (n.d.). Back Safety and Safe Lifting. Retrieved from https://www.uah.edu/images/administrative/facilities/oehs/back_and_lifting_safety_secured.pdf

74. MHI. (n.d.). The Ergonomics of Manual Material Handling: Pushing and Pulling Tasks. Retrieved from http://www.mhi.org/media/members/14023/130258038292642021.pdf

75. UNC. (n.d.). Lifting and Material Handling. Retrieved August 21, 2019, from https://ehs.unc.edu/workplace-safety/ergonomics/lifting/

76. Knapik, G. G. and Marras, W. S. (2009). Spine loading at different lumbar levels during pushing and pulling. *Ergonomics, 52*: 1, 60–70. doi:10.1080/00140130802480828. http://dx.doi.org/10.1080/00140130802480828

77. Shoulders, M. D., & Raines, R. T. (2009). Collagen structure and stability. *Annual review of biochemistry, 78*, 929–958.

78. Elliott, B. (2018, April 06). Top 6 Benefits of Taking Collagen Supplements. Retrieved August 21, 2019, from https://www.healthline.com/health/collagen-powder-benefits

79. McKenzie, R (2011). *Treat Your Own Back*. Spinal Publications New Zealand Ltd. Raumati Beach, New Zealand.

80. Miller, R. (2003, May 14). Avoid Back Injury with the Right Lifting Techniques. Retrieved August 23, 2019, from https://www.spine-health.com/conditions/sports-and-spine-injuries/avoid-back-injury-right-lifting-techniques

81. Celis-Morales, C. A., Lyall, D. M., Welsh, P., Anderson, J., Steell, L., Guo, Y. et al (2017). Association between active commuting and incident cardiovascular disease, cancer, and mortality: Prospective cohort study. *Bmj*. doi:10.1136/bmj.j1456

82. Step Jockey. (n.d.). The Health Benefits of Stair Climbing Challenges. Retrieved August 23, 2019, from https://www.stepjockey.com/health-benefits-of-stair-climbing

83. Jung, J. H., & Moon, D. C. (2015). The effect of thoracic region self-mobilization on chest expansion and pulmonary function. *Journal of physical therapy science*, *27*(9), 2779-81.

84. Pahwa R., & Jialal, I. Chronic Inflammation. [Updated 2019 Jun 4]. In: StatPearls [Internet]. Treasure Island (FL): StatPearls Publishing. Available from: https://www.ncbi.nlm.nih.gov/books/NBK493173/

85. Harvard Health Publishing. (2006, April). Inflammation: A unifying theory of disease. Retrieved August 23, 2019, from https://www.health.harvard.edu/newsletter_article/Inflammation_A_unifying_theory_of_disease

86. Hamer, M., Sabia, S., Batty, G. D., Shipley, M. J., Tabák, A. G., Singh-Manoux, A., & Kivimaki, M. (2012). Physical activity and inflammatory markers over 10 years:

follow-up in men and women from the Whitehall II cohort study. *Circulation*, *126*(8), 928–33.

87.   Terry, G. C., & Chopp, T. M. (2000). Functional anatomy of the shoulder. *Journal of athletic training*, *35*(3), 248–55.

88.   Julius, A., Lees, R., Dilley, A., & Lynn, B. (2004). Shoulder posture and median nerve sliding. *BMC musculoskeletal disorders*, *5*, 23. doi:10.1186/1471-2474-5-23

89.   Ohio State University. (2014, August 15). Addressing The High Corporate Costs of Back Pain (and other MSDs). Retrieved August 23, 2019, from https://spine.osu.edu/blog/2014/08/addressing-high-corporate-costs-back-pain-and-other-msds

90.   Saint-Maurice, P. F., Troiano, R. P., Matthews, C. E., & Kraus, W. E. (2018). Moderate-to-Vigorous Physical Activity and All-Cause Mortality: Do Bouts Matter? *Journal of the American Heart Association,* *7*(6). doi:10.1161/jaha.117.007678

91.   Heneghan, N. R., Baker, G., Thomas, K., Falla, D., & Rushton, A. (2018). What is the effect of prolonged sitting and physical activity on thoracic spine mobility? An observational study of young adults in a UK university setting. *BMJ open*, *8*(5), e019371. doi:10.1136/bmjopen-2017-019371

92.   Page P. (2012). Current concepts in muscle stretching for exercise and rehabilitation. *International journal of sports physical therapy*, *7*(1), 109–19.

93.   Di Cagno A, Minganti C, Quaranta F, Pistone EM, Fagnani F, Fiorilli G, et al. Effectiveness of a new cervical pillow on pain and sleep quality in recreational athletes with chronic mechanical neck pain: a preliminary comparative study. *J Sports Med Phys Fitness* 2017, 57:1154–61. DOI: 10.23736/S0022-4707.16.06587-7

94.   Mayo Clinic Health System. (2017, March 8). Poor posture can cause shoulder pain. Retrieved August 7, 2019, from https://mayoclinichealthsystem.org/hometown-health/speaking-of-health/poor-posture-can-cause-shoulder-pain

95. Nakamura, K., Kodama, T., & Mukaino, Y. (2014). Effects of active individual muscle stretching on muscle function. *Journal of physical therapy science, 26*(3), 341–344.

96. Wickstrom, B. M., Oakley, P. A., & Harrison, D. E. (2017). Non-surgical relief of cervical radiculopathy through reduction of forward head posture and restoration of cervical lordosis: a case report. *Journal of physical therapy science, 29*(8), 1472–1474.

97. Martarelli, D., Cocchioni, M., Scuri, S., & Pompei, P. (2011). Diaphragmatic breathing reduces exercise-induced oxidative stress. *Evidence-based complementary and alternative medicine : eCAM, 2011*, 932430. doi:10.1093/ecam/nep169

98. Asher, A., CPT. (2019, April 28). Info on the Transverse Abdominus Muscle That Influences Core Strength. Retrieved August 7, 2019, from https://www.verywellhealth.com/transverse-abdominal-muscle-297289

99. Cleveland Clinic. (2018, September 14). Diaphragmatic Breathing. Retrieved August 7, 2019, from https://my.clevelandclinic.org/health/articles/9445-diaphragmatic-breathing

100. Rodriguez-Merchan E. C. (2014). Evidence Based Conservative Management of Patello-femoral Syndrome. *The archives of bone and joint surgery, 2*(1), 4–6.

101. Kiecolt-Glaser J. K. (2010). Stress, food, and inflammation: psychoneuroimmunology and nutrition at the cutting edge. *Psychosomatic medicine, 72*(4), 365–369. doi:10.1097/PSY.0b013e3181dbf489

102. Harvard Health Publishing. (2008, December). Treating osteoporotic fractures of the spine. Retrieved August 7, 2019, from https://www.health.harvard.edu/newsletter_article/Treating_osteoporotic_fractures_of_the_spine

103. National Research Council (US) Steering Committee for the Workshop on Work-Related Musculoskeletal Injuries: The Research Base. Work-Related Musculoskeletal Disorders: Report, Workshop Summary, and Workshop Papers. Washington (DC):

National Academies Press (US); 1999. Response of Muscle and Tendon to Injury and Overuse. Available from: https://www.ncbi.nlm.nih.gov/books/NBK230857/

104. I-Min Lee, MBBS, ScD; Eric J. Shiroma, ScD; Masamitsu Kamada, PhD; David R. Bassett, PhD; Charles E. Matthews, PhD; Julie E. Buring. (2019). Association of step volume and intensity with all-cause mortality in older women. *JAMA Intern Med*;179(8), 1105-1112.

105. Lavey, R., Sherman, T., Mueser, K. T., Osborne, D. D., Currier, M., & Wolfe, R. (2005). The Effects of Yoga on Mood in Psychiatric Inpatients. *Psychiatric Rehabilitation Journal, 28*(4), 399–402.

106. Wells, M.E., Vaughn, B. (2012) Poor Sleep Challenging the Health of a Nation. *The Neurodiagnostic Journal* .Volume 52(3), 233-249.

107. Depner, C.M., Stothard, E.R. & Wright, K.P.(2014) *Current Diabetes Reports* 14: 507.

108. Esposito, K., Giugliano, D., (2004) The metabolic syndrome and inflammation: association or causation? *Nutrition, Metabolism and Cardiovascular Diseases.* 14(5), 228-232.

109. Witvrouw, E., Mahieu, N., Danneels, L. et al. (2004) *Sports Medicine.* 34(7), 443-449. https://doi.org/10.2165/00007256-200434070-00003

About the Author

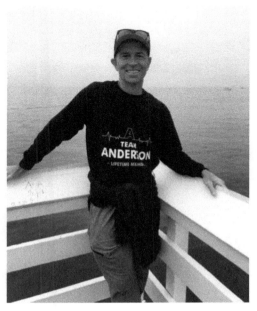

Dr. Parley Anderson is a native Nevadan, born in Las Vegas and raised in Pahrump. After graduating from Pahrump Valley High School, Parley moved to Reno and has lived here for the last twenty-five-plus years. Parley attended the University of Nevada, Reno, where he earned a BS in education and then studied fitness management in Grad School. During his time at UNR, Parley taught Personal Health and Lifestyles and also directed the university's fitness center. Anderson then attended the University of the Pacific, where he earned both a master's and doctorate in physical therapy. Parley has been a practicing physical therapist for the last 17 years, 15 of them in private practice ownership. His office (Active Physical Therapy) is located in Caughlin Ranch at the corner of West Plumb and West McCarran (3594 West Plumb Lane). Additionally, Parley is a professor of kinesiology and has been teaching at the University of Nevada for the last ten years. Parley is also a strong advocate for his profession, having served in a variety of professional volunteer positions, including two terms as president of the Nevada Physical Therapy Association. Besides being a physical therapist, Dr. Anderson is also a certified CrossFit instructor.

CPSIA information can be obtained
at www.ICGtesting.com
Printed in the USA
LVHW070821121120
671500LV00010B/541